Your Reiki Treatment

Your Reiki Treatment

Bronwen and Frans Stiene

Founders of the International House of Reiki

info@reiki.net.au
www.reiki.net.au

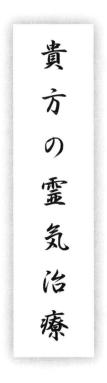

貴方の霊気治療

BOOKS

Winchester, U.K.
New York, U.S.A.

First published by O Books, 2007
O Books is an imprint of John Hunt Publishing Ltd.,
The Bothy, Deershot Lodge, Park Lane, Ropley,
Hants, SO24 0BE, UK
office1@o-books.net
www.o-books.net

Distribution in:

UK and Europe
Orca Book Services
orders@orcabookservices.co.uk
Tel: 01202 665432
Fax: 01202 666219 Int. code (44)

USA and Canada
NBN
custserv@nbnbooks.com
Tel: 1 800 462 6420
Fax: 1 800 338 4550

Australia and New Zealand
Brumby Books
sales@brumbybooks.com.au
Tel: 61 3 9761 5535
Fax: 61 3 9761 7095

Far East (offices in Singapore, Thailand,
Hong Kong, Taiwan)
Pansing Distribution Pte Ltd
kemal@pansing.com
Tel: 65 6319 9939
Fax: 65 6462 5761

South Africa
Alternative Books
altbook@peterhyde.co.za
Tel: 021 447 5300
Fax: 021 447 1430

Text copyright Bronwen and Frans Stiene 2007

Design: Jim Weaver

ISBN-13: 978 1 84694 013 2
ISBN-10: 1 84694 013 3

A CIP catalogue record for this book is available from the
British Library.

Printed in the US by Maple Vail

CONTENTS

PREFACE

There are many warm and open hearted people who have been involved in the creative process of writing *Your Reiki Treatment*. We must always begin with offering thanks to our families as they are the foundation of our world. Our mothers and our daughter, Bella, are always there for us; reaching out and catching us, restoring us and simply loving us for who we are.

There are many case studies in *Your Reiki Treatment*. The majority are based on our experiences with clients and students. Clients' names have been changed to maintain their privacy as well as events and even circumstances where necessary. At the same time we have retained the thematic purpose at each case study's heart in order to educate the reader. Some case studies have not been personally experienced by us but have been reported by fellow practitioners or clients and are therefore anecdotal. The intent behind their inclusion is to highlight problems that a client may face either with a practitioner or in a specific Reiki treatment situation.

Thank you to our students and clients who constantly teach us about the experience of Reiki and have provided us with the knowledge and expertise required to produce *Your Reiki Treatment*.

Our podcast interviews from *The Reiki Show* have been an amazing inspiration. Without that tool we would never have met so many motivated, surprising and wonderful individuals. Your words, and often generosity, have made a great impact upon us, more than we had ever imagined possible. Thank you. A special mention to those who have provided information relevant to *Your Reiki Treatment*: Julie Anderson, Angie Buxton-King, John Coleman, Sue Lake-Harris, Phyllis Lei Furumoto, Doreen Sawyer, Mari Stevenson, Kansaku Yosei, Pamela Miles and Graham King.

Thank you to the many open-hearted individuals who have helped the book writing process. This includes:

Akhila Hughes for her editing, down-to-earth advice and friendship. Reverend Jion Prosser for the set of four beautiful kanji that are spaced throughout *Your Reiki Treatment* and for his kindness. Li Ying for her energetic support, wisdom and friendship. All of our teachers, past and present. And a big thank you to everyone at O Books who have helped to make *Your Reiki Treatment* a reality.

Some of the organizations whose processes have provided information for *Your Reiki Treatment* are the Australian Reiki Connection (ARC), the Council of Australian Reiki Organisations (CARO), the UK Reiki Federation (UKRF), the UK Reiki Regulatory Working Group (UKRRWG), and the National Center for Complementary and Alternative Medicine (NCCAM).

Thank you, too, to the many ethical and caring researchers studying biotherapies in order to bring attention and respect to the ancient art of healing in whatever name or guise it may hold.

May this book bring pleasure and support to all clients and practitioners of the system of Reiki everywhere.

> Managaichi ayamariga arimashitara goyousha kudasai
> Please forgive us if we've made a mistake

INTRODUCTION

The system of Reiki has had many varied incarnations since its quiet beginnings as a spiritual practice in Japan in the early 1900s. By the late 1920s some of the teachings had evolved into a healing treatment called Usui Reiki Ryôhô and was practiced by Japanese naval officers. This soon developed into the first professional Reiki clinic, run by Hayashi Chûjirô. In the 1930s it traveled across the sea to Hawaii where it took on a new life as Reiki, a healing system practiced by Mrs Takata. She remained its head in the West until she passed on in 1980. It was at this juncture that the system was given a makeover and became a New Age trend which has included at various times chakras, spirit guides, extraneous levels and exciting, yet questionable, histories. It continues to be taught in Japan today as a mix of the old and the new.

Moving forward into the 21st century, the system of Reiki is gradually leaving a disparate past and cottage industry label behind to take on its latest role as an integrative therapeutic treatment that is headed toward being openly welcomed in hospitals around the world. At the same time the teachings are reconnecting with their spiritual roots in the Japanese culture and philosophy, rounding the practice off as a therapy of substance; one that is gaining a foothold in mainstream society's vocabulary, minds and hands.

Reiki practitioners have studied the system of Reiki in order to help themselves, friends, family and colleagues with treatments at home, at work and occasionally as paid practitioners in a clinic. As governments and communities call for clearer guidelines regarding the composition of therapies today, a new therapeutic face within the system of Reiki is emerging – the Professional Reiki Practitioner. This new practitioner has been searching out suitable role models and relevant teachings to define who and what she is and how she can most effectively fulfill this title. She has the skills, ability and confidence to work full-time in this role in her own business or within a larger clinic or hospital environment.

Add to this equation another new face, the Professional Reiki Client – you. You come to a Reiki treatment with the expectation of receiving a professional treatment colored by your previous experiences with other health care services.

Together, the professional practitioner and client have been determining the boundaries of what it means to receive a professional Reiki treatment. This unfolding of a clearer definition of a professional Reiki treatment has also found support and guidance in various arenas from relevant associations and Reiki schools to government agencies. It is an exciting development that also signals change for many Reiki practitioners who have been practicing to their own drumbeat and may now need to alter their rhythm to fit with that of a clearer understanding of the system of Reiki in its professional setting.

Your Reiki Treatment focuses on the client's experience before, during and after a professional Reiki treatment. The client is the vulnerable ingredient in this promising formula and needs to be fully informed of any risks or possible consequences in order to feel relaxed and confident and to receive the most from a Reiki treatment.

In the first Part of *Your Reiki Treatment*, Pre-Treatment, you are assisted in finding and choosing an appropriate Reiki treatment. You also learn about practitioners, venues, fees, treatment variations, Reiki for pregnancy, children, pets, and using Reiki with those suffering from specific illnesses such as cancer and depression.

Part II, The Treatment, dissects the experience of a Reiki treatment. The procedure, the length of the treatment, the practitioner's process, your sensations during the treatment, and everything that transpires up until the last moments of your session as you walk out the clinic door.

Your treatment continues after leaving the clinic and this is covered in Part III, Post-Treatment. It is possible that your body will begin to cleanse itself both physically and non-physically and practical techniques are described to help you move through this process at home. Also included is additional information about the system of Reiki and its relationship with other practices, as well as some revelations about the state of Reiki research today.

This wider acceptance of therapies such as Reiki as a professional health care choice has been called the Silent Health Care Revolution[1]. The rapid rise of complementary and alternative medicine (CAM) usage over the last 10 years is changing the face of health care. Reiki is commonly listed as CAM under the branch, biotherapy. Reiki has not yet, however, received full support in some health care sectors. Certainly, the concept of self-responsibility and self-healing as promoted by the system of Reiki can be a difficult concept to grasp for a health industry that has various motivations – many humanitarian, yet some damaging.

Looking positively, research undertaken in 2006 shows that 57% of physicians felt that incorporating CAMs into their practice would have a positive effect on client satisfaction. Also 44% stated that they would refer their clients to a CAM practitioner if one was available at their institution. However, physicians also felt that randomized, controlled trials were the minimum level of evidence required for CAM provided at their practice.[2]

Throughout *Your Reiki Treatment* a number of conclusions from research papers are included to satisfy this need for scientific evidence. It incorporates research relating to relevant integrative therapies, including Reiki, and their efficacy with treating those with cancer, pain, etc... These studies support the modern mind's understanding of what a Reiki treatment is and how it works.

Correspondingly, also included are the more esoteric understandings of Reiki: a system that promotes preventative health care and spirituality in the one breath as well as supporting you in finding inner balance and balance within your natural environment.

The better grasp that society has on a system such as Reiki, the more willing it will be to accept that these values and principles are fundamental to living healthy and contented lives.

Your Reiki Treatment aims to support the move toward a common standard of Reiki education for both clients and practitioners. In this new world the myths that have hovered around the fringes of the system of Reiki are dispelled, the clients' and practitioners' roles and boundaries are straightforward, and everyone is assisted in getting the best out of this profound energetic practice.

Although there are different legal obligations for different countries regarding professional therapies, there are certain standards within the system of Reiki that are global. *Your Reiki Treatment* will be invaluable to the global professional Reiki clients and practitioners by offering them benchmarks to work with. It intends to be a reference point that is both familiar and executable.

How to read this book:
- Each chapter can be read individually or you can read *Your Reiki Treatment* in its entirety.
- Find your relevant chapter with ease due to the consistent chapter length.
- Enjoy the case studies, research, client tips or Reiki myths by flicking though *Your Reiki Treatment*.
- A glossary has been included to support your understanding of Japanese words and any Reiki related language that you may be unfamiliar with.

The contents of this book are for general information only. The authors accept no liability for the use or misuse of any practice or technique in this book.

Japanese pronunciation:
a is similar to the **a** in father
i is similar to the **ea** in eat
u is similar to the **oo** in look
e is similar to the **e** in egg
o is similar to the **o** in go

An Introduction to Modern Japanese
Osamu and Nobuko Mitzutani

Part I

Pre-Treatment

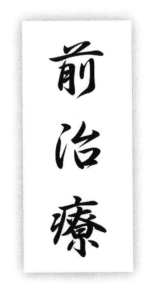

REIKI: THE NON-INVASIVE THERAPY

The system of Reiki is unique, which explains why it has become the model for many contemporary energetic forms of healing. It offers a simple structure of three levels of study for those wishing to learn it and after training at that first level it is possible to offer Reiki treatments to friends and family. Once the second level is completed, and the Reiki practitioner has gained treatment experience, it is possible to begin treating clients professionally.

Reiki is the energy that moves through your body, in fact Reiki practitioners understand that Reiki is the energy that moves through everything and is often called universal life force energy. During a Reiki treatment a practitioner supports the movement of this energy within your body, yet doesn't manipulate it.

Healing with Hands a Reality

The energy fields projected from the hands of bodyworkers are in the range of intensity and frequency that can influence regulatory processes within the body of another person.[3]

All aspects of your existence are interconnected. When you experience healing it is not just one aspect of yourself, but many small and interconnected aspects, that are moving back into balance with one another. At this point your body is alleviated from the stress, pain, or dysfunction that you were experiencing.

You, too, are one of those interconnected aspects of your community, and your community is an interconnected component of your culture, and that culture interconnects with other cultures to create the world that you and your friends and family live in. Once you become more balanced, your friends may also become more balanced, and then the domino effect of good health will be repeated throughout the networks within your community, culture and eventually your world.

Furthermore, this interconnectedness occurs not just at the human level. In nature, plants, animals and insects, the mountains, rivers and plains – all interconnect with humanity to create a healthy, balanced cosmos. The quality of your existence begins with you. Once you create this healthy balance within yourself, you are ready to fit together with another balanced piece of the puzzle. Together, your healthy relationship starts to make sense and everything around you begins to fall into place.

Each step that you take on the grass, each sip of water, each breath of air, and each whiff of a flower's perfume is you interacting and creating a relationship with the world around you. You nurture the grass, the water, the air, the flowers so that they may support and pleasure you. These connections that you constantly create are your healing landscape – you are a part of this landscape.

Not many people know what to expect at their first Reiki treatment. It is in many ways a strange experience as communication between the client and practitioner takes place, for the most part, energetically with no diagnosis being given. This is far removed from the experience of visiting a doctor or even most natural therapists.

A Reiki treatment is therapeutic, rather than diagnostic, in that it aims to support a client's self-healing and well being – not alleviate any particular diagnosed illness.

Usui Mikao's Description of Reiki in Relation to Modern Science

My method is beyond a modern science so you do not need knowledge of medicine. If brain disease occurs, I treat a head. If it's a stomach ache, I treat a stomach. If it's an eye disease, I treat eyes. You don't have to take bitter medicine or stand for hot moxa treatment. It takes a short time for a treatment with staring at the affected area or breathing onto it or laying on of hands or stroking with hands. These are the reason why my method is very original.

Reiki Ryôhô Hikkei
Usui Reiki Ryôhô Gakkai

WHERE TO FIND A REIKI TREATMENT

There are a number of avenues available to you when searching out a suitable Reiki practitioner. You will be seeking someone you feel comfortable with, who works professionally, and who is experienced as a practitioner.

The best place to start is by asking someone you know. This might not sound like a particularly professional approach, yet in the relatively short time that you spend on the Reiki treatment table your eyes may be opened to elements of yourself that you would not normally recognize. A Reiki treatment feels personal, not because it is in any way invasive or manipulative or even diagnostic, but because during a treatment you may be awakened to new or unusual experiences or feelings.

For this reason you need to feel comfortable and confident and not concerned about the actions of your practitioner. The more confident and comfortable you feel, the more effective your treatment will also be.

Word-of-mouth will point you in the direction of a recommended practitioner, one who has satisfied or fulfilled a previous client's expectations. Therefore, there is a reasonable chance that this will also occur for you. Ask around at work, with your friends or your family.

In your search for a professional practitioner, if you have had no luck through word-of-mouth, you can look at paid advertising. This might be in the local telephone directories, health and healing magazines, online advertising or on professional Reiki websites. To find a local website type the words "Reiki treatment" plus the name of your city or region into a search engine.

Generally, if a practitioner is buying advertising it means that she is earning money through her Reiki treatment practice, indicating a minimal level of experience. Paid advertising, however, says nothing about the practitioner's ethics or level of energetic expertise. Beware of Reiki practitioners claiming to use more effective Reiki techniques than others, who have secret methods, or who offer cures – these attitudes are not acceptable within the system of Reiki and are not a reflection of a professional Reiki practitioner.

An avenue you can try is to approach an association or accrediting body. In this situation you need to be aware of the standards of the association or body. Some may refer practitioners who have satisfied specific entry criteria and continue to maintain a high level of professionalism. Another so-called association may simply be an entity that lists its own graduating students with no true professional standards in place.

It is quite common for notices from local Reiki practitioners offering their services to be found on bulletin or notice boards at Health Food stores, in libraries, natural therapy centers and in community centers.

Where to Find your Reiki Treatment

- Word-of-mouth.
- Bona fide industry associations.
- Internet websites.
- Magazines in health food stores.
- Bulletin/notice boards in community centers.
- Bulletin/notice boards in libraries.
- Bulletin/notice boards at natural therapy centers.

No matter where you find the contact details of a Reiki practitioner, it is always wise to make contact with the practitioner prior to arriving at your Reiki treatment. You can do this by simply having a chat on the telephone, but you do need to make sure that this person will be providing a service that you feel will be beneficial for you. To indicate what you are likely to experience during a Reiki treatment you can ask the practitioner a number of pertinent questions.

Questions to Ask Practitioners

As Reiki treatments grow in popularity on a global scale, many people will admit to knowing the word Reiki but few can tell you exactly what it means or what a treatment entails. There are many varied, and sometimes contradictory, ideas about the system of Reiki and how a Reiki treatment should be performed. This is quite common with energetic therapies that have undergone continuing adjustment by individual teachers and practitioners over time. Reiki treatments can, therefore, be performed in a number of ways but it is the many commonalities between all Reiki treatments that will be addressed within the pages of *Your Reiki Treatment.*

As the client, you are in a position where you can ask as many questions of the Reiki practitioner as you wish. The practitioner's answers will help you decide if the practitioner and his particular style of treatment is what you are looking for. Here are some questions that might help you find the treatment that will serve you best.

Initial Questions to ask your Practitioner

- Q. Where is the treatment held?
- Q. What are your hours?
- Q. Do I need to make an appointment?
- Q. What is the length of a treatment?
- Q. What does it cost?
- Q. What is your background?
- Q. What is your cancellation policy?

Once you have asked these basic questions, it is time to start probing into the finer details of the practitioner's method of treatment.

- ***Q. What is involved in a Reiki Treatment?***
Listen to the practitioner's explanation and see if what the practitioner explains is acceptable to you. As a client you have full rights to state that you do not want something or do not wish certain

practices to occur. Does the practitioner sound confident and professional? – if not, then avoid placing yourself in a vulnerable position and telephone the next practitioner on your list.

- **Q. Do you do anything else apart from Reiki practices during your treatment and do you have professional indemnity insurance?**
Some practitioners may include massage, aromatherapy, psychic or spiritual readings, reflexology or other practices in their Reiki treatments. Legally, Reiki treatments are not considered high risk as there is no physical manipulation involved. Including other therapies into a treatment may raise this level of risk. If these non-Reiki practices are not what you require, ask if you can receive a treatment without them. If this is not possible then pull out your practitioner list and get back on the telephone. Professional practitioners will always have professional indemnity insurance.

- **Q. How long have you been practicing professionally?**
With this question you can find out about the practitioner's professional energetic experience. A professional practitioner should ideally have worked in a supervised setting to perfect his understanding of Reiki treatments before beginning work as a practitioner.

THE PRACTITIONER'S QUALIFICATIONS

The system of Reiki is moving into a new era. Initially, the system was introduced to the West from Japan by Hawayo Takata in the late 1930s and any form of regulation of the system of Reiki was held in her grasp until she died in 1980. She was a petite, first generation American with Japanese parents who was considered a strict teacher by her students. Many of those students were also awed by her charisma and assuredness. After her death there was a period where the system of Reiki began to unravel which was likely due to a lack of infrastructure – in spite of the efforts of some. For a time the name, Reiki, came to mean any number of practices from Native American Indian visualizations to Tibetan chants.

Now, more than 25 years later, the system is attempting to rediscover its basic commonalities and Japanese roots in order to integrate with the changing regulations facing complementary and alternative medicine from governmental agencies. Nationally recognized accreditation systems and voluntary self-regulation are becoming a fait accompli for the system of Reiki in a number of countries.

The global networking capabilities of the internet effectively ensure a wider understanding of what it means to practice Reiki today. This may at times confuse and dumbfound but can also provide the opportunity to further support Reiki research and encourage communication between practitioners.

The unraveling has therefore slowed enormously and many teachers, organizations and associations are attempting to role the ball back into some sort of comprehensive shape. This can only bode well for the future of the system of Reiki.

For Reiki clients it implies the expectation of a higher quality of industry professionalism with, as bare minimum, professional Reiki practitioners holding insurance and membership with bona fide associations. Such organizations offer practitioners accepted standards and codes to enable them professional status in the eyes of insurance companies and often the general Reiki industry. Organizations provide certification that denotes a practitioner's level of membership and will be on view at the Reiki clinic along with any other relevant qualifications that a professional practitioner may hold.

Reiki industry standards generally require that a professional practitioner hold at least a Level II certificate qualification. However, in some countries, a Level I certificate is accepted as a professional qualification if the practitioner can show treatment experience and ongoing personal development with Reiki and relevant techniques. If a Reiki practitioner offers counseling, massage or any other therapy, it is wise to ensure that the practitioner is actually qualified to do so before accepting treatment in this field.

Qualifications are a part of modern society and have been put in place to protect clients but they have very little to do with the quality of Reiki that clients receive. To cover this important aspect of your Reiki treatment, you can ask your practitioner about her own self-healing regime. The level of development and personal wellbeing of a Reiki practitioner are also integral to your treatment as this following research shows.

In Vitro Effect of Reiki Treatment on Bacterial Cultures: Role of Experimental Context and Practitioner Wellbeing

Objective: To measure effects of Reiki treatments on growth of heat-shocked bacteria, and to determine the influence of healing context and practitioner wellbeing.

Results: For practitioners starting with diminished wellbeing, control counts were likely to be higher than Reiki-treated bacterial counts. For practitioners starting with a higher level of wellbeing, Reiki counts were likely to be higher than control counts.

Conclusions: The initial level of wellbeing of the Reiki practitioner correlates with the outcome of Reiki on bacterial culture growth and is key to the results obtained.[4]

In reality, as far as the efficacy of your Reiki treatment goes, the proof is in the pudding. You will only know how effective the treatment is once you have experienced it.

QUESTIONS ABOUT YOUR
PRACTITIONER'S QUALIFICATIONS

Due to the fact that qualifications are a contemporary requirement, here are some questions that you can ask your Reiki practitioner to ensure that you will be receiving the Reiki treatment you had expected.

• *Q. Are you a Level II practitioner or a teacher?*

Level I in the system of Reiki teaches a practitioner how to use Reiki for healing on herself, and on friends and family. The focus at this level should be largely on the self and not on others, however it is beneficial for a practitioner to experience working on others in a non-professional environment at this stage. Once a practitioner has developed energetically and completed Level II, he may become a professional practitioner. For the client it does not matter whether the practitioner has a Level II or teacher certificate (sometimes called Level III, Shinpiden, Master or Master/Teacher certificate) as it is the practitioner's energetic experience and professional skills that will dictate the quality of the treatment. Be aware that with some Reiki training it is possible for a practitioner to learn Level I and II together. This standard is largely unacceptable within the Reiki industry as the practitioner has had no opportunity to gain energetic experience between levels.

• *Q. Are you currently a member of a bona fide Reiki association?*

If the practitioner is a financially paid up member of a bona fide association and is registered by that association as a professional practitioner you have some level of assurance of the quality and professionalism of the practitioner. A practitioner should have a certificate confirming these facts on display. A code of ethics should also be available to the client along with a complaints procedure, if so requested.

- **Q. Do you have any professional qualifications apart from your Reiki certification?**

In some countries new regulations are being developed where practitioners can receive accreditation as professional Reiki practitioners with nationally recognized organizations. Apart from a practitioner requiring the minimum of a Level II certificate in the system of Reiki, the accrediting board may also require the completion of training in communication skills, Occupational Health and Safety, First Aid, basic knowledge of anatomy and physiology and business skills. It is advantageous if a practitioner continues to upgrade his skills both practically and theoretically in order to ensure ongoing high quality treatments inline with current standards are provided.

- **Q. Please tell me what the system of Reiki means to you? Has it changed you in any way?**

These questions are aimed to draw the practitioner out on subjects relating to his own experience with Reiki. They are not about paper qualifications, but personal ones. From this question you will learn how he became involved with Reiki, which area of Reiki he is passionate about and what type of self-healing regime he practices (if any). To understand why self-treatment is important, imagine that a practitioner is a garden hose. If there are many knots and kinks in that garden hose, only a small dribble of water can trickle from it. By undoing these knots and kinks, the water is free to rush out with full force. If the practitioner is not actively undoing his own knots then only a trickle of energy can move through him. If, however, the practitioner constantly works at undoing these knots, the energy is free to flow in abundance and the client can draw all the energy needed.

Whether a practitioner is a Level II or III is unimportant as far as your treatment goes. It is not the name that the practitioner is using (eg. Reiki Master) that is important but the quality of the practitioner's energetic experience.

The Treatment Room

In reality a Reiki treatment can take place anywhere – in an office, park, bathroom, lounge room, or bus – all that is required is two individuals: the client and the practitioner.

For a professional treatment to take place, however, the Reiki practitioner must create a space that is conducive to healing while offering a professional service.

A practitioner's treatment room may be at home in a specially outfitted room or it may be in a clinic with other therapists who offer a wide range of natural therapies that may include massage, acupuncture or aromatherapy. These days it is even possible to receive Reiki from practitioners working in doctor's surgeries. Another venue for a professional practitioner to work from is in a hospice, hospital or community center – in the current climate this is still commonly viewed as a voluntary position, but is gradually changing. And lastly, some practitioners may even be able to visit you with a mobile Reiki treatment practice.

What to Expect in the Treatment Room

- A clean, quiet and private place where you will not be interrupted and confidentiality is ensured.
- A room temperature that is neither too warm nor cold.
- Somewhere to sit where you can discuss the treatment with your practitioner prior to, and after, the treatment.
- An adjacent washroom.
- A comfortable treatment table that you can access with ease.
- An alternative to a treatment table such as a comfortable chair, depending upon your personal requirements.
- A light blanket in case your body temperature lowers during the treatment.

The more welcoming the venue, the more relaxed you will feel and the greater the opportunity to heal. If you enter a comfortable room with soft music and a friendly practitioner, you are prepared for your healing to begin. A sense of safety ensures your openness to the experience ahead of you.

Relaxing music is optional, as are candles. Although a practitioner may find that candles are atmospheric, some clients may find such an environment foreign or too intimate. For this reason a practitioner should always be aware that she does not take the ambience too far. Many clients enjoy and almost expect relaxing music to be played during a Reiki treatment today. Some clients have even been known to bring along their favorite CD.

Naturally, these optional extras may not be acceptable in a hospital or hospice and therefore it is good to know that they are merely optional rather than a requirement. If a client in a hospital wishes to listen to relaxing music a practitioner might provide headphones and a music player – this can be beneficial to help clients remove themselves mentally from the hospital environment which may not always be conducive to healing.

It is important to realize that ultimately a treatment is what you make of it. As a client, if you do not feel comfortable then it is necessary that you inform the practitioner that aspects of the venue are unsuitable. The practitioner should be open in supporting you with this or you should take the step of finding yourself a more suitable practitioner.

Choosing a Venue that Supports your Healing

Grace entered the Reiki treatment room at her local natural therapy center and immediately felt uncomfortable. She was confronted with a menagerie of religious icons that were foreign to her own beliefs. Lining the walls was what she called "new age memorabilia" including a pyramid collection, crystals and candles. Grace paid the same price for her Reiki treatment as she did for her regular massage at the same center. For this reason she had expected an environment that reflected the same standard of professionalism and respect for her beliefs. After her Reiki treatment Grace thankfully returned to her regular massage therapist.

Choosing a Student Clinic

Some Reiki training centers offer clients the choice between a student clinic Reiki treatment and a professional Reiki treatment. A student clinic is where a Reiki student performs a treatment under the supervision of a teacher. The industry standard generally requires that this student should already have completed Reiki Levels I and II. A student clinic treatment is naturally a cheaper option and is excellent for those who wish to "taste" a treatment or for someone who is chronically ill and may require long-term treatments.

A Reiki treatment might appear to be a simple procedure due to the fact that it does not utilize diagnostic procedures. However, there are two major areas that your Reiki practitioner needs to excel in. One is in energetic experience, where he must learn how energy works, and the other is in the practicalities of professional treatment delivery where he studies what it means to be a professional therapist. A student clinic works at increasing a student's proficiency in these two areas.

When beginning to study the system of Reiki a practitioner focuses first on the self to develop a clear understanding of what energy means and what its side-effects are. The Japanese founder of the system of Reiki is quoted as saying that, "If you can't heal yourself, how can you heal others?"[5]

To ensure that the client feels safe and confident a teacher must be present throughout the treatment. If the client is uncertain about the student's competency then the full benefit of the Reiki treatment cannot be experienced. The less open a client and practitioner relationship, the less successful the treatment. The teacher's presence also allows the teacher to assess the student's treatment for discussion at the end of the clinic session.

Lessons at a Student Clinic

John welcomed his client, Annie, at the door. This was John's first client at the student clinic and he was careful not to show that he was feeling nervous. After just five minutes of working with Reiki on Annie's head, her limbs began to quiver and then shake involuntarily. John's confidence disappeared and his hands began to waver. Fortunately, John's teacher who had been sitting quietly in the room came over and assessed the situation – Annie's eyes were still closed and she seemed unperturbed by the erratic movements. He indicated quietly that John should continue with the treatment, which he did. Gradually the shaking subsided as John moved from the head down to the torso. After the treatment Annie told John that she felt fantastic; she'd never felt so relaxed. She'd been totally unaware of her shaking limbs! John was relieved that he had not interrupted the treatment unnecessarily and that he had allowed Annie's body to release whatever it needed to.

It is also necessary that practitioners learn clear communication skills, how to dress appropriately, create an ambient atmosphere in the clinic, how to take client case studies professionally, and even how to request payment for services rendered.

Clients can therefore expect a high quality treatment from a student clinic. Students are generally dedicated and serious, occasionally more so than some self-proclaimed professional practitioners.

As a client you will want to know if the energy is as strong and effective from a student as it is from a professional. It is true that the more a practitioner works on himself the more energy can move through him to be available for the client's healing. It is, however, impossible for anyone to gauge this strength, it is totally subjective. Energetic expertise is totally unique to each individual with practitioners naturally having their own energetic strength and balance to begin with. All that is known is that the more you work at it, the more effective it becomes. Remember too, that even though some people may call themselves professional practitioners, they may have neglected to develop themselves energetically.

DISTANT TREATMENTS

A distant Reiki treatment is where a healing technique is performed by a Reiki practitioner on a client who is not in the practitioner's physical vicinity. The client could be in the next room or in a country on the other side of the world. There should be no difference in the quality of this unique form of treatment no matter how far the distance between the practitioner and client in physical terms.

Level II Reiki practitioners study techniques for connecting energetically to clients with the intention that the clients will draw on that energy to heal themselves. The energetic concept is exactly the same as an in-person Reiki treatment.

In the distant healing technique the practitioner visualizes or senses the energy of the person she is going to perform a Reiki treatment on. She may use tools to create a supportive environment for this process. A photo of the client, for example, can help the practitioner develop a stronger energetic sense of the client. The practitioner then moves into a meditative state and connects with the client on an energetic level, allowing the client to draw on the Reiki.

A client may sense this energetic offering. It is not necessary to know that you are receiving a distant Reiki treatment but if your awareness is with the experience then there is a chance that you may be more open for healing to take place. For this reason many Reiki practitioners discuss with the client an exact date and time for the distant treatment to occur in order to support the client's experience.

A Reiki practitioner is taught that when she is performing a treatment, either in-person or from a distance, her intention is to offer Reiki in order that the client may take what she needs at that exact moment in time. A practitioner should never try to manipulate, or dictate the energy. Naturally, it would be disrespectful to attempt to offer Reiki when a potential client has categorically stated that she does not want a treatment. In such a circumstance the client will most likely not draw on the Reiki as she is not open to it.

The more experienced the practitioner is at self-healing and working with a distant healing technique, the more effective the process will be.

Although distant Reiki treatments work energetically in much the same way as regular Reiki treatments do, for a number of reasons it may be preferable to have an in-person Reiki treatment. Touch and a listening ear are healing stimulants and an in-person Reiki treatment, unlike a distance treatment, provides these wonderful tools. The illusiveness of distant healing means that you can never be sure that the treatment has been performed as promised. Therefore you may wish to entrust the practice of a distant treatment to a practitioner you know or one who has been recommended to you.

There are times when distant Reiki treatments might be more suitable than in-person treatments. Perhaps it is possible that you are unable to access a Reiki treatment or you may request healing for a family member who is sick.

Online distant healing networks where you request healing are often free – just type *distant healing* into the search engine. Many training organizations have networks or *absent healing books* where the client's name can be added to a list and Reiki Level II and III practitioners regularly perform distant treatments for those individuals.

Professional practitioners may also include distant treatments as a service though not necessarily for free. If you are required to pay for a distant treatment, gauge the cost of the treatment by the length of physical time that the practitioner spends on the distant treatment. When you pay for a Reiki treatment you are not paying for the energy but for the practitioner's time, experience and professionalism.

TREATMENT FEES

The cost of a Reiki treatment may indicate the quality of a treatment but that is, as with everything in life, not always the case. Treatment fees will depend upon a number of variable factors. This means that you cannot expect consistent pricing between Reiki practitioners.

To begin with you will need to take into consideration the length of time of the session. Many sessions are one-hour in length, though it is also possible to experience shorter and longer sessions often depending upon the practitioner's training guidelines. Naturally, you are paying for a professional's time.

Depending upon the practitioner's level of training and expertise, the cost will also vary. Some practitioners may have many years of hands-on experience, while some may have completed training in various styles of Reiki, complementary therapies and supportive forms of professional development.

A professional has his own fees to pay including the hire or rent of the venue. Insurance, association fees, taxes plus the cost of materials and advertising are just some of the additional expenses that a practitioner must recoup from the treatment fee to maintain a viable business.

A question that has been raised in the past – should a Reiki treatment cost anything at all? Isn't universal energy free?

Yes, it is – but the constraints of this life insist that we use money as a means of exchange to buy food and shelter. For this reason it is naturally appropriate that you pay for the time and expertise of a professional. One thing to remember though – you can never pay for Reiki itself. It is impossible to pay for energy.

Not only must we respect and give thanks for the energy, but the same applies for the role of the practitioner.

It is respectful in any culture, modern or ancient, to give thanks for the efforts of one who supports us. There is no less intention of love if one requests payment for services rendered. In fact, the services are more likely to be enacted in a professional manner and may include the practitioner having experienced diverse Reiki training and having trained in counseling, Occupational Health and Safety, First Aid and much more.

It is up to you, the client, to decide how much you wish to pay for a Reiki treatment and then look for a treatment that is within that price range. It may be with a highly experienced practitioner or in a student clinic. Remember, the most important aspect of healing is that you are comfortable and therefore capable to open up to heal. A large part of your healing experience centers upon you.

Non-professional practitioners may not ask for money if they are helping friends and family, with their financial overheads being few, if any. To offer a treatment in this manner can be very satisfying for the practitioner as he experiences a sense of helping others.

THE PRACTITIONER'S INFLUENCE ON YOUR TREATMENT

From the first moment that you make contact with your Reiki practitioner she will influence you – that is human nature. This same natural law also ensures that you will influence your practitioner.

How you influence each other and what you take to, and away from, your shared experience is something that you both have control over.

Your practitioner can influence you through her looks, words, actions, and attitude. A Reiki treatment is safe, non-invasive and non-manipulative, the only danger that it can pose is when a practitioner forgets her duty of care to the client. Ethically, one of the basic concepts of any therapy is respect for the client's autonomy. A practitioner must hold a client's safety and individual rights uppermost in her mind at all times.

Your Client Rights

It is fundamental to a just and ethical society that people are autonomous and able to control their bodies and what others are permitted to do to their bodies. It is for the client, not the practitioner, to determine if and when any procedure or treatment should occur.

Complementary Medicine: Ethics and Law
Michael Weir

The practitioner's attitude toward how Reiki itself works will also greatly affect the client and the outcome of the treatment. Reiki may incorrectly be seen as a tool for the practitioner rather than the practitioner being a tool for the energy to move through. A practitioner who believes that the energy is a tool, something to "use" for healing or spiritual growth, is one who believes she is in control of the energy. This can lead to a practitioner diagnosing or judging what is best for the client, which in itself can lead to an attempt on the practitioner's behalf to offer an undue influence on the client. This is not considered to be beneficial or ethical for either party.

Reiki works at all levels of our human experience. It is not solely logical or physical in nature, it is a holistic system. Deciding what is right or wrong for a client is not working holistically or with the client's best interests at heart. A Reiki practitioner is not trained to advise clients on their health status; energetic matters are subtle and advice concerning them is inappropriate. For example, if a practitioner tells a client that her energy is blocked then the client may come to believe this and experience serious issues (some even physical) relating to the practitioner's energetic diagnosis. Energetic diagnosis is entirely subjective.

As a client it is important that you feel empowered throughout your Reiki treatment and that you ensure that the practitioner's influence is a positive one. A client may decide at any time before, during or after a session that the practitioner's duty of care has been unsatisfactory. It should be reasonable for a client to ask questions of the practitioner at any time. This is where you can influence the session by constantly taking up your right of choice. Your choices are numerous: Is your practitioner a woman or a man, close to your home or a train ride away, in a clinic or at her home, what does she charge? Every step of the way there are choices for you to make and you must make these in an ongoing effort to remain empowered, ensuring you receive the best treatment possible. Intimidation or bullying exercised by a practitioner in a treatment environment is unacceptable and indicates a lack of duty of care.

TREATMENTS WITH MORE THAN ONE PRACTITIONER

It is possible to have a Reiki treatment with more than one Reiki practitioner. This may sound a little kinky at first but be assured it is absolutely above board.

Receiving a treatment from more than one practitioner at any one time is often called Group Reiki or Shuchu Reiki. This means that two, three or even more people will place their hands on, or near, your body during a Reiki treatment.

This is a wonderful experience, although there is a possibility that first-time clients may find it overwhelming. Many hands on the body can unearth ingrained fears and clients need to be aware of their own boundaries and not be shy to voice their thoughts if they feel at all uncomfortable.

Getting use to Touch in a Safe Environment

At the beginning of Justine's Level I Reiki course she openly stated that she did not wish to be touched at all. Fortunately, Reiki can be performed without touching the body and everyone respected Justine's wishes. On the first day of the course Justine's practice partner performed an entire Reiki treatment on her with hands slightly off the body – not touching. The next day, when the students merged into groups to practice Group Reiki, Justine surprised everyone by being the first to jump up on the table. She then encouraged her group of four to *make sure* they put their hands on her body. Now that the Reiki from the first day of the course had supported her in moving through her concerns relating to touch in a safe environment, she was ready to experience Reiki at its, arguably, most enjoyable.

A professional practitioner would never offer Group Reiki to a client without first informing the client prior to the treatment. Reasons for offering Group Reiki might be that the practitioner is teaching students in a student clinic environment and the treatment is performed together. Once again, a client should be informed of this prior to the treatment.

In contemporary western societies we do not touch very often – a peck on the cheek as we leave, or arrive, at our relatives' homes, and a hug when we are feeling in the mood for warmth and connection are often all that we experience. This western model of independence may well be the reason for Reiki's popularity. Booking yourself in for an hour of touch once a week is a wonderful antidote to an insular world. Touch is integral to an ongoing healthy existence and a Reiki treatment addresses that.

Is Group Reiki more effective than one-to-one treatments? It can feel very cocooned and loving to receive Group Reiki. This is naturally beneficial and will enhance a client's openness to the treatment. Yet, there is no proof that states it is more effective. The most influential person in a Reiki treatment is always you – the client. It is you who draws the energy, and it is you who heals.

PREPARING YOURSELF MENTALLY

Reiki treatments are unique because you, as a client, play a major role in the success of the treatment.

Although the concept of healing today may be portrayed as one of luxurious pampering – this is just one aspect of a Reiki treatment. Yes, the environment might be attractive, the music soothing, the Reiki practitioner professional and kind but the real responsibility behind the success of the treatment lies with you.

The more open that you are to your Reiki treatment the greater its effect. A Reiki practitioner simply creates the space for your healing to take place. It is you, albeit largely unconsciously, who draws on the Reiki to clear your body of obstacles in an effort to achieve a state of equilibrium.

You can support this process by preparing yourself mentally for your treatment. Clearly set your thoughts, this is called your *intent*, to know that during your Reiki treatment you will receive whatever it is that you need at this particular moment in your life. Such a clear intent allows for deep healing to take place as you have set no limit upon what you may receive. If you were directing the energy, you would be working largely with the rational mind which is unable to hear the true voice of the whole you.

Your relationship with everything depends on your intent. If you set the intent that you receive whatever you may need at this exact moment in your life then the healing will go much deeper than if you try to direct it. It will become easier to leave behind impure intentions when you focus on allowing the healing to take place rather than trying to manipulate it. These continued actions will lead to your intent becoming clearer and more effective.

Support your Healing by learning this Maxim off by Heart:

I am open to receive whatever it is that I may need at this exact moment in my life.

Ultimately, how you imagine your life is how you experience it. Everyone has ups and downs but it is your perspective, your intent, which is the true creator of your reality.

Everything is Universal Energy

Patrick had spoken to a couple of different practitioners prior to his Reiki treatment trying to find out how it would work and if there was anything that he needed to know or do to make the treatment more successful. One Reiki practitioner told him a number of unfounded superstitions. He told Patrick that a Reiki practitioner could not wear black or red clothing or any jewelry at all, and that the practitioner must be a non-garlic eating vegetarian, otherwise the energy would not flow properly. Patrick felt correctly that the practitioner was not grounded and went and booked a treatment with someone else. Unfortunately, the superstitions did concern him and made him question what was appropriate. When he walked in the door and saw the practitioner's black shirt he wondered if his treatment would be unsuccessful.

Patrick needed to know that everything is made of universal energy and therefore the superstitions *were* totally unfounded. His uncertainty had made him less open for a healing experience. The practitioner put fear into Patrick's mind – a very unethical practice and one that should never be associated with Reiki. This fear set Patrick up to have beliefs about the system of Reiki where no beliefs are required.

EXTRA PREPARATION CONSIDERATIONS

Do you need to change your diet, stop smoking or refrain from wine to ensure the success of your Reiki treatment?

If you do any of the above quite suddenly you are most likely going to cause yourself a great deal of consternation and stress and create more problems than you had when you began to walk this path.

Ideally, the move to change your current situation should evolve naturally, without force. By forcing yourself, you will only encourage further imbalance. If there is a time for you to leave smoking and drinking behind or to change your diet, Reiki will assist that process naturally. This is a much healthier attitude to work with, rather than trying to operate to the beat of another's drum and forcefully stopping in order to receive a Reiki treatment.

To experience Reiki, and for it to be effective, it is helpful if you understand that Reiki is not something outside of yourself. It is even possible to say that you are Reiki. Energy is a part of you and is constantly moving through you, it is not as if you are separate from the universe – you are a part of it.

The Universe is You

Universal energy created the sun, the moon and the earth, and created the ocean on the earth and bred the creatures from there and evolved mankind. Universal energy exists even in the weeds as well as in a single grain as Life energy. Human life exists also as a part of Mother Nature (the universe).

Modern Reiki Method for Healing
Doi Hiroshi

With Reiki you accept *more* energy into the body and it begins to work away at any areas that may be stagnant. Reiki will support you in changing your lifestyle and you will find that this may be quite subtle in nature.

You are in Control

Pete was 28 and slightly concerned that these Reiki treatments, which he was enjoying, would affect his party-going lifestyle. His girlfriend, Danielle, had tried a Reiki treatment first and she had loved it so much she had convinced him to try it out. After his first treatment on a Friday afternoon he'd decided to take the night off and relax quietly at home instead of meeting with friends at a local club. A similar thing had happened after his second treatment where, although he did go out this time, he really didn't feel like drinking at all. Curiously, he was also feeling good in himself but at the same time he was a little tentative that Reiki might be stirring up greater changes than he was prepared to make. Pete began to understand that there was no cause for alarm; he could stop with the Reiki treatments if he wanted to or he could continue and allow the change to occur naturally in its own time – it was his choice and he was now, more than ever, in control of his life.

As you now know, when you receive a Reiki treatment, the intent held by both you and your Reiki practitioner is that you will receive what you need at this exact moment in your life. Nothing will occur that is not sanctioned by you, even at an unconscious level. Yes, change may be on its way but it is with your permission.

All that you can do to prepare yourself is to chose a practitioner that you feel is right for you, wear something that you feel comfortable in and make sure you are on time. Reiki will take care of the rest.

REIKI AND PREGNANCY

It is completely safe to receive a Reiki treatment when pregnant as long as the Reiki practitioner exercises responsible duty of care. She must ensure that you are comfortable and relaxed. There are special treatment tables available that have been developed to fit a pregnant woman's shape or alternatively a comfortable chair is also suitable. Sitting in a chair in no way inhibits the movement of energy.

Naturally, it is not only the mother that is receiving the Reiki treatment but also the baby. Many mothers experience that their baby settles during a treatment and heaviness in the uterus can be felt due to this. Other mothers state that it stimulates the child. In this way, it is once again apparent that Reiki treatments are individual to the client, even if the client is a baby growing inside her mother's body.

When a mother-to-be receives a Reiki treatment, the practitioner asks her to focus on the Reiki maxim that she will receive whatever it is that she and her baby need at that particular moment of their lives. The practitioner then sets the same intent for the mother and baby.

Connecting with your Baby

Mary arrived at her Reiki treatment with only three weeks to go before her due date. She had felt tired and emotional prior to the treatment but afterward she said she felt wonderfully relaxed and so much more connected to her baby. During the treatment the baby had settled and she felt that it was very relaxed. Mary wanted to be able to repeat the experience at home and the practitioner recommended that in a quiet moment she simply place her hands on her baby with the intent to offer energetically whatever the baby needed. She also recommend that Mary return a week later for another treatment as further support. Mary returned the next week, amazed. Each day she had placed her hands on herself and her baby and they had both become wonderfully relaxed.

Some Reiki practitioners will not perform Reiki treatments on pregnant women. This indicates that the practitioner is inexperienced and lacks a comprehensive understanding of how Reiki works. Practitioners will often suggest to pregnant women and their partners that they learn how to practice Reiki themselves in order to encourage an energetic connection within the family long before the baby is even born.

Once your child enters the world you can continue with this wonderful practice. Not only does it assist developing your connection together, it is a required element for your child's growth.

Supporting your Child through Touch

More recent studies suggest that during formative periods of brain growth, certain kinds of sensory deprivation – such as lack of touching and rocking by the mother – result in incomplete or damaged development of the neuronal systems that control affection.

The Origins of Human Love and Violence
James W. Prescott, Ph.D.

TREATING CHILDREN

Touch is something we continue to enjoy and even crave through-out our lives, often long after society might believe that we "need" it. The uniqueness of touch is a quality that soothes and appeases our often overworked nervous systems.

As with any health care service that a child attends, a guardian must always be present throughout the entire session. Depending on local legislation the age will vary as to how old a child may be to consent to receiving a Reiki treatment. Some regions permit minors over the age of 16 years to consent to medical treatment and although this does not relate directly to complementary and alternative medicine it provides an indication of what is a minimum appropriate age for valid consent.[6] Not only is it a legal requirement to gain consent for the treatment of a child but the child will feel much safer, and therefore more open to healing, when a guardian is present.

Children and Mental Health Care

In the USA, 21% of children aged between 9 and 17 receive mental health care services in a given year.[7]

This statistic validates the need for the introduction of additional health care services such as Reiki which are non-intrusive, em-powering and can support children through their life changes and challenges. Children need help to deal with this world and parents can often be at their wits end finding ways to assist them. Many Reiki practitioners have commented that the introduction of simple Reiki practices into schools could go a long way to supporting entire communities.

A child's treatment may also take place on a treatment table. How-ever, a younger child does not necessarily have the patience to lie, or even sit, for almost an hour and for this reason a practitioner will approach a child's treatment differently to that of an adult. A Reiki practitioner creates a treatment that supports a child's needs.

Children will quite bluntly tell you whether they think they would like a Reiki treatment or not. Listen to the child. Forcing anyone to have a Reiki treatment works against one of the five Reiki Precepts: *For today only be compassionate to yourself and others.*[8] Although children might be less experienced in practical terms within the world, energetically they may well be more in touch with themselves than an adult. If you learn to trust your child's wisdom, that child's confidence will soar and your connectivity will grow in leaps and bounds. You are nurturing a child who will instinctively understand what he needs, unfazed by societal demands – a rare quality.

Therefore, make sure you consult your child first about the idea of experiencing a Reiki treatment. Perhaps the child can meet with the practitioner prior to the treatment where a brief explanation of how Reiki is given and may even be experienced.

Children can be very open to energy and may have a direct experience of their connection with the universe and may see bright lights or darkness. The immediateness of these experiences could possibly be frightening. For this reason the practitioner should always discuss the treatment with the child either during and/or after the treatment to ensure that there are no concerns left in the child's, or parents', minds to take home. A good practitioner will be able to clearly explain the child's experience to the whole family.

The wonderful saying, 'Children learn to smile from their parents' acknowledges that a child is a reflection of his parents. Always take a long, careful look at yourself first when your child is unwell. Perhaps it is you, your partner or someone in your child's close environment who should also be receiving a Reiki treatment. Parents and children are always encouraged to learn Reiki together – it broadens the family's understanding of life and brings everyone closer together as they share the joy of Reiki.

TREATING PETS

Curiously, pets are a little like children with their lack of pretension. A pet will either accept a Reiki treatment or not.

Animal Reactions to Reiki

///

Animals are much more sensitive than humans to energy in general and feel Reiki energy immediately and strongly. Many animals will startle or stop in their tracks when they first feel Reiki energy.

///

Animal Reiki
Elizabeth Fulton and Kathleen Prasad

The length and nature of a pet's Reiki treatment will depend upon each individual animal. Some animals will lie or sit comfortably allowing the practitioner to place hands on, or near, the body for as long as the animal's body draws the energy. An animal's Reiki treatment will generally consist of simply placing the hands directly at the site of the complaint. This does not mean that the entire treatment is necessarily short. A Reiki practitioner needs to take time to get to know your pet, make friends and offer the energy before beginning the actual treatment.

Even Animals need Time to Work through Life's Challenges

Jessie became a street dog after losing her owners. She hunted through garbage for her food and ran frightened in between the traffic. One day, she found herself in a cage where she was given food, though little attention and she was surrounded by dogs in cages. Jessie felt like she had lived her whole life in fear. A family with two children came to her cage one day. They talked to her and petted her and then chose to take her back home with them. She loved her new family but always had this feeling in the back of her mind that they may one day leave her behind.

Her family thought Reiki would help Jessie's nervousness, but whenever the practitioner offered Jessie Reiki she whimpered and moved away. The sensation of Reiki, of energy moving in the body, was unpleasant and stirred things in Jessie that she did not want to face. Jessie's owners had to accept this and the practitioner felt that what Jessie needed most of all was lots of love and then maybe one day in the future Jessie would feel confident enough in her life situation to face more Reiki.

It is often easier for a practitioner to come and visit your pet at home rather than your pet having to travel to a strange treatment venue. In the home environment your pet may feel more relaxed and open to healing.

You can also request that the practitioner send Reiki to your pet using a distant healing technique. Distant treatments do not require your pet to be physically present for the procedure. The practitioner needs to be able to energetically connect with your pet and may often use a photo of your pet along with a description which may include, name, age and complaint.

A professional practitioner may also recommend that the pet's owner study how to work with Reiki. This is a wonderful resource for any animal that requires healing. Just like you, your pet has many layers to work through in this lifetime and any support you can offer is a true gift.

Looking after the Both of You

If your pet needs Reiki why don't you make sure you receive a Reiki treatment too? It will help you to be calm and support your pet in her time of need. Some people believe that pets take on illnesses for their owners. If this is the case then looking after yourself will certainly be looking after your pet too.

CONTRAINDICATIONS TO REIKI

In earlier chapters the safety of a Reiki treatment has been discussed in relation to pregnancy, children and even pets.

Reiki is a safe practice that can only ever harm when a Reiki practitioner neglects to offer appropriate duty of care. If the practitioner's venue is unsafe or the practitioner offers unqualified advice or treatments then duty of care has been breached. Duty of care includes elements such as a practitioner being aware if his client requires emergency medical attention at any time during the Reiki session.

Reiki will change how you feel, think and behave – if you let it. This is you finding a renewed balance in your life and that cannot be harmful.

A competent, professional practitioner will keep full records of the Reiki session. Within these records will be a client record form with the client's details plus a section alerting the practitioner to any medication that you may be taking. At this juncture the practitioner will explain that Reiki is energetic in nature and relies to a large degree on you, the client, to draw energy into your body. This can often be sensed and may produce a natural clearing called the cleansing process.

As Reiki works not only on the physical body but also on your emotional and spiritual aspects, then your clearing may affect all facets of your life. This clearing is not a contraindication to Reiki and yet a client needs to be made aware of how a natural healing process functions. A clearing can mean that you experience an extra high or low after a treatment, that your conditions become temporarily worse before they improve, or you may find that you come down with a cold, a headache, or diarrhea.

A clearing is viewed as a positive experience even though the temporary "symptoms" may not be pleasant. By allowing your body to remove its own imbalances you have initiated and supported your own self-healing; a therapeutic and empowering process.

Your own Natural Pharmacopoeia

//

Each of us has his or her own natural pharmacopoeia – the very finest drugstore available at the cheapest cost – to produce all the drugs we ever need to run our bodymind in precisely the way it was designed to run over centuries of evolution. Research needs to focus on understanding the workings of these natural resources – our own endogenous drugs – so that we can create the conditions that will enable them to do what they do best.

//

Molecules of Emotion
Candace B. Pert, Ph.D.

For many people this is a totally new paradigm and yet when you begin to live it, you discover that it is true – the human body can heal itself.

Other effects experienced from a Reiki treatment relate to your medication. It is possible that changes in your current wellbeing due to a Reiki treatment may positively affect the levels of medication you currently require. There is anecdotal evidence that diabetics, for example, have found that their medication requirements alter when receiving Reiki treatments. Naturally, you must never self-medicate and always discuss any changes to prescription medication with your doctor.

REASONS TO CHOOSE REIKI

A Reiki practitioner may never claim to be able to cure an illness. No scientific evidence exists that can uphold such an assertion. This claim is also not in line conceptually with the system of Reiki. A Reiki practitioner simply allows each client to fulfill their own healing journey. Healing may include a full spectrum of outcomes from miraculous healing to humanity's final outcome in a peaceful death. The philosophy behind the system of Reiki is that death is a part of the human journey and that Reiki can support us not only in living but also in dying. Anecdotally, it is accepted in the Reiki community that no matter the state of your physical condition, whether you are in excellent health or living with disease, Reiki can still aid you in its ability to bring about balance. This assists you in feeling peaceful and accepting, regardless of your physical condition.

The system of Reiki is a practice that, although it does not diagnose, manipulate or offer products to a client, is considered as effective as many other respected therapies today. It relies on the wisdom of the body to know what it needs and wants, in contrast to the controlling and often unempowering attitude of other invasive health care practices. There is a great wisdom underpinning this system as it teaches its practitioners to leave their limited rationality behind, hold on tight to their commonsense, and let the world's natural flow of healing energy run its course.

Achieving Deep Healing without Intellect

Certainly, for those who use their hands to enhance the functioning of their fellow beings, the 'free-run' periods, when allowed to happen without intellectual processing, can give rise to moments of profound insight and deep healing.

Energy Medicine: The Scientific Basis
James L. Oschman.

Quackwatch founder, Stephen Barrett MD, has deemed Reiki "worthless" along with other therapies such as massage. His reason for stating this is that it has not been scientifically measured and therefore "it doesn't exist." He did admit that it may make you feel good but that, in itself, had no effect on cancer or the immune system. [9] Research today sees this differently – especially research relating to the placebo effect and human responses to the environment.

It is true that the scientific community, which has the ability to measure infinitesimally small units of matter, finds the concept of ancient and traditionally accepted terms like Ki, prana or chi difficult to grasp. There have been mixed results from research largely due to these difficulties. Is it because they are looking in the wrong direction, trying to measure Reiki in the same way that they would a new pill on the market? Today there are numerous Reiki studies taking place across the planet, all with the aim to measure the effect of Reiki and many, perhaps more practicably, are attempting to measure the client's response to Reiki.

It is research in the latter area that has resulted in a reasonable degree of success. This is because it is possible to gauge a client's sense of wellbeing by asking questions of the client. A sense of wellbeing, contrary to Stephen Barret MD's comments, has many implications for a client's health. It appears that a Reiki treatment can provide "an overall improvement in both quality of life and symptom distress"[10] in clients with diseases.

The Effects of Less Anxiety and Stress

Numerous studies show that eradicating anxiety and stress ... would, in itself, greatly increase longevity and decrease illness.

The Biology of Transcendence
Joseph Chilton Pearce

The system of Reiki is a holistic system. Not because it tells you what to eat, wear, or do but because of its understanding that everything is interconnected. How you feel and what your attitude to life is, can all make a difference to the quality, and perhaps the longevity, of your existence. The system of Reiki works at this level with each individual, validating life as a profoundly spiritual and meaningful experience.

USING ALCOHOL AND DRUGS WITH REIKI

Can you be under the influence of alcohol and/or drugs when you receive a Reiki treatment and still experience its benefits? The first point that should be made is that a Reiki practitioner has the right to refuse a client a Reiki treatment if the client is under the influence of alcohol and/or drugs. These substances can invalidate a treatment and, more importantly, a client under the influence may create an unsafe environment for both the practitioner and the client.

To explain the invalidating effects of alcohol and drugs on a treatment, imagine yourself as more than just a physical being – you are also an energetic one. You are a being that is filled with Reiki. When you experience a Reiki treatment you draw more energy into your body. This works at clearing your energetic pathways, bringing you gradually into a balanced state. A balanced state refers to a state where everything in your body is functioning well: your liver is sending bile to your gall bladder, your brain is directing messages coherently through its central nervous system, and your emotions are neither diving nor peaking due to a balanced hypothalamic-pituitary-adrenal axis. Reiki supports this natural need for your body to work effectively. Drugs, however, confuse the body. They affect your natural healing abilities and mask the true needs of your system. Your body loses its inner wisdom and is unable to function in a balanced manner.

Drugs Confuse your Healing System

///

Drugs, legal and illegal, are further interrupting the many feedback loops that allow the psychosomatic network to function in a natural, balanced way, and are therefore setting up conditions for somatic as well as mental disorders.

///

Molecules of Emotion
Candace B. Pert, Ph.D.

When you receive a Reiki treatment and your body's signals are confused and unable to communicate, one would imagine that the energy you draw, if you can draw it at all, will spend most of its time trying to find a way out of the maze that it is in. For this reason there is likely very little benefit in receiving Reiki while under the influence of alcohol and/or drugs. The struggle is harder and it is wiser, in order to gain the most from your treatment, to attempt to be in a state of openness.

Interestingly, it is wise to remember that there will always be obstacles for the energy to work with, whether the client is under the influence of alcohol and/or drugs or not. A client who is completely conscious and energetically clear is an enlightened being – in a perfect place of balance – and this state, though ideal, is uncommon (if not non-existent) in clients. This means that even if you are not under the influence, energy will move through you inefficiently. By continuing to work further on yourself with Reiki you will find that this begins to improve with time. Your energetic pathways become stronger and more able to accept larger amounts of energy through you, offering a more balanced experience of life. The difference between attending a Reiki treatment under the influence of alcohol and/or drugs and being in a regular state of imbalance is that you have made a deliberate choice to inhibit the effectiveness of your treatment by being under the influence. This intent is a conscious attempt to block your healing process.

You will not harm yourself if you receive a treatment while under the influence of alcohol and/or drugs unless, for example, you are at such a point of incapacitation that it is impossible for you to lie on a table safely. Nowadays, Reiki treatments are offered at many outdoor festivals where patrons have access to, and enjoy partaking in, what some may call social drugs. Although receiving a treatment in such an environment is not ideal, a Reiki treatment cannot be harmful under such circumstances. However, whether it is beneficial is another matter entirely.

REIKI FOR CANCER

Scientists have been researching the relationship between a patient's energy field and the onset of cancer for many years.

Back in the 1930s Harold Saxton Burr stated that:

> ... diseases would show up in the energy field before symptoms of pathology, such as tumors.[11]

This was confirmed in 1987 when a study showed that:

> ... the conductance changes in tumors are highly frequency dependant. Direct measurements showed 6.0-7.5 times higher conductances in tumors compared to normal tissues (Smith et al 1986). In later stages of both cancer and AIDS, tissues begin to deteriorate and electrical conductances drop."[12]

Finally in 1996, Brewitt also stated that:

> ... disease states can be detected by measuring changes in the electrical conductances of tissues making possible early diagnosis and treatments."[13]

James L. Oschman cites these studies and more, and concludes that life force has not been ruled out as a form of healing in modern research. Bioenergy fields, he believes, have gone from scientific "nonsense" to a new and developing subject of biomedical research. Today, the system of Reiki is commonly listed as a biofield therapy. He goes on to state that cancer is a whole system phenomena that cannot be understood by examining parts rather than relationships. Therefore, looking at just the cancer is not the pathway to prevention or cure. Further research into this discovers that the body has a correct, or healthy, frequency. This healthy frequency is what we often refer to as being in a state of balance. James L. Oschman describes the body's physiological processes (which are all interconnected and linked) as the regulation of a whole system. According to this collection of research, diseases such as cancer may first become apparent energetically rather than physically. If this can be dealt with and brought back into balance before the physical body is affected, a system such as Reiki could be an effective preventative practice. A Reiki practitioner can sense when the body's energy is more active in specific organs or regions. She does not diagnose but allows the body to draw energy through that area until a sense of balance or calm is realized. She then moves to the next position on the body where energy is active and drawing. These basic actions of a Reiki practitioner when put in the light of modern research may well be a vital preventative measure.

The Brownes Cancer Support Centre *2004 Patient Care Report* stated that its services were primarily used by women (85%) with almost half having breast cancer. Reiki was the most accessed treatment from all the therapies on offer. The report's conclusion was that there was an overall improvement in both quality of life and symptom distress scores for patients. There was also an improvement in these areas over the course of the sessions from treatment 1 to 6.

Another study published in *Integrative Cancer Therapies* in 2003 by Dr Post-White used healing touch with cancer patients in a randomized trial. Results showed that a relaxed state was induced, with lowered respiratory and heart rates and lower blood pressure. The therapies also reduced short-term pain, mood disturbances and fatigue.[14]

Healing takes place at many levels as everything you are, and experience, is interrelated. To maintain a high quality of life it is recommended that you access quality foods, adequate sleep, experience low stress levels, and address your attitude to life. Reiki is not something separate from you – it is in you, your environment, your friends and the food you eat. Coming into balance using Reiki is to come into balance with your world.

REIKI FOR STRESS AND DEPRESSION

Most people at some point in their lives experience stress and/or depression to varying degrees.
Stress may be external or internal. External stress comes from your environment or relationships. This may include work stress which the World Health Organization has stated is a worldwide epidemic. It also includes energetic stress from the ever growing number of computers, microwaves, and mobiles that you deal with everyday. Internal stress comes from psychological issues where you may "worry yourself sick" for example. Depression may be triggered by major life changes like birth, death, and divorce.

Stress and Depression

- 80% of workers feel stress on the job.[15]
- 14% of respondents had felt like striking a co-worker in the past year, but didn't.[16]
- 25% have felt like screaming or shouting because of job stress.[17]
- 18.8 million American adults suffer from clinical depression. That is 9.5% of the adult population.[18]
- Anxiety disorders, as a group, are the most common mental illness in the US. About 40 million American adults are affected by these debilitating illnesses each year.[19]

Stress plays an important role in the functioning of your system: it readies you for the danger that is approaching. To do so it affects your heart and blood vessels, immune system, lungs, digestive system, sensory organs and brain. Extreme stress may cause fear, short-term memory loss, and may affect your rational thought. This general stressing of your body therefore affects you both physically and emotionally. Over the long-term this may also result in any number of symptoms such as pain or depression when a client cannot process the stress or feels a lack of control due to the constant stress that is experienced. In fact, stress has been said to be linked to the six leading causes of death – heart disease, cancer, lung ailments, accidents, cirrhosis of the liver, and suicide.

Reiki practitioners feel that Reiki can be effective in calming the body and alleviating stressful symptoms. Current research appears to support these claims.

Long-term Effects of Energetic Healing on Symptoms of Psychological Depression and Self-perceived Stress

Objective: To study the long-term effects of energetic healing.

Trial: Six participants were randomly assigned to one of three groups: hands-on Reiki, distance Reiki, or distance Reiki placebo, and remained blind to the treatment condition. Each participant received a 1-1.5 hour treatment each week for 6 weeks.

Results: Upon completion of treatment, there was a significant reduction in symptoms of psychological distress in treatment groups as compared with controls (P < .05; Eta square ranging from .09-.18), and these differences continued to be present 1 year later (P < .05; Eta square ranging from .12-.44).[20]

Although a client may begin to feel more whole and balanced from receiving Reiki treatments, he must not stop taking any prescribed medication unless advised to do so by his physician. Reiki can be utilized as a preventative measure for stress by helping clients re-balance and find a center of peace within before a possible escalation into serious physical or emotional imbalance occurs.

Stress: the Killer

A landmark 20-year study conducted by the University of London concluded that unmanaged reactions to stress were a more dangerous risk factor for cancer and heart disease than either cigarette smoking or high cholesterol foods.[21]

REIKI FOR ENLIGHTENMENT

An enlightened state is one where there is a unique awareness of existence; to hold an understanding of the perfection of yourself within the perfection of the universe and to act in accordance with that.

A Reiki treatment takes a step up to the doorway of enlightenment. During the treatment a thread is further developed and strengthened between you and the greater universe. When you walk that thread you are offered a glimpse, a very brief and fleeting one, of an awakened awareness that could be yours. In that moment a realization of possibility is tantalizingly dangled in front of you. If you have the possibility to know it once, you have the possibility to know it again and again until the state becomes one of permanence.

This sampled sense of enlightenment may feel like you are very light or as if you are interconnected with everything around you. To analyze what this sense is or what brought it about is unnecessary. It is an experience that should be seen as an encouragement to continue with additional inner healing. Of course, enlightenment is not realized in a one-hour treatment, it is a lifetime journey.

Inherently, you are a free flowing, clear river of energy without any obstructions. During your lifetime you gradually take on obstructions: bad experiences you haven't dealt with, good experiences you are too attached to, societal perceptions, your own judgments and much more. Burdened by these obstacles, your river can no longer run free and clear. With Reiki you begin to purge yourself of these hindrances, by drawing on more energy to wash them away. Your aim is to return to the state where your energy can run free again and return to your true nature – Reiki assists you with that.

The link between healing and enlightenment is that the more Reiki you receive the more your programmed thoughts and prejudices are released, opening you up to remembering your true connection to life and everyone and everything within and without that realm.

What a Bitch!

Megan had been receiving Reiki treatments for a number of weeks and was really starting to feel their benefits. She believed she was now less stressed, calmer and more aware of her life choices. The ultimate realization of how true this was occurred when her work colleague approached her with these jaw dropping comments: "You're so much more fun to work with these days. It's great that you're not as bitchy any more. Believe it or not, I'm actually enjoying coming to work at the moment." Megan was stunned. Had she been that difficult to work with? Megan had not only helped herself by receiving Reiki treatments but apparently her actions had unintentionally helped improve the lives of those around her.

Working with Reiki produces a ripple effect. Your inner change can be the instigator for change in your outer environment, affecting everyone and everything.

A wonderful aspect of the system of Reiki is that there is no dogma attached to it. It can easily be incorporated into any religion or practice that holds specific beliefs without interfering with them. It can also easily be added to your own spiritual practice whether that be meditation, yoga, qi gong etc... Practitioners on a spiritual path will, as with any journey, find that there are times when the practice moves with ease and other times where the road is bumpy or apparently impassable. Reiki can be an excellent adjunct that moves you through these difficult times to support your main practice and even help you move deeper into it. Reiki has a high level of compatibility due to its profound simplicity.

A Great Teaching

These are truly great teachings for cultivation and discipline that agree with those great teachings of the ancient sages and the wise. Sensei named these teachings 'Secret Method to Invite Happiness'.

Usui Mikao Memorial Stone
Saihōji Temple, Tōkyō

REIKI AS FIRST AID

In the 1920s, Japan was emerging as an industrial nation with western culture affecting many aspects of Japanese life. Still relatively untouched by these changes was the Japanese medical profession. Many traditional Japanese healing practices were still in use. There was also, at the time, a general attraction to the concept of hands-on healing (called *teate* or *tenohira*).

A number of Japanese naval officers were attracted to the hands-on-healing aspects of the system of Reiki. These naval officers were members of a society called the Usui Reiki Ryôhô Gakkai, which still exists in Japan today. It is believed that they first began learning Reiki in order to help themselves and their fellow servicemen while out on their vessels. Reiki would have worked preventatively aiding the sailors in feeling calm and relaxed in their confined environment. It is also believed that Reiki was used as a form of First Aid. The Japanese word *teate* can also be translated to mean a form of First Aid.

Historical use of Reiki for Healing

Ki and light are emanated from the healer's body, especially from the eyes, mouth and hands. So if a healer stares, or breathes on, or strokes with hands at the affected area such as toothache, colic pain, stomachache, neuralgia, bruises, cuts, burns and other swellings – the pain will be gone.

However, a chronic disease is not easy, it needs some time. But a patient will feel improvement at the first treatment.

Reiki Ryôhô Hikkei
Usui Reiki Ryôhô Gakkai

The wonderful benefit to using Reiki as a form of First Aid is that no matter where you are there is one tool you will always have with you – your hands. In a crisis hands, placed on a wound, a panicked head or a broken limb, will help calm the situation and at the same time support the system in coming around to a point of balance.

Anecdotal evidence from Reiki practitioners claims that blood is stemmed, calm is invoked and pain is relieved when hands are brought into First Aid situations. More and more studies are being conducted into the efficacy of Reiki in an effort to support its vast amount of traditional evidence.

A research paper, *The Use of Reiki in Psychotherapy*, concluded that clients reported an overall experience of warmth, wellbeing and safety that seemed to diminish pain and heighten awareness.[22]

Reiki is obviously not comparable to, or to be used solely instead of, First Aid today but it is there to support you in times of acute need. If you fall over, for example, a by-stander may offer Reiki to you. This may reduce the degree of bruising, pain or emotional discomfort that may have resulted from your accident. You just need to be willing to accept the healing, even if it is while you are lying on the pavement waiting for the ambulance to arrive.

Reiki in a First Aid Situation

Jeremy's son, James, had fallen off his pushbike and had a long, deep cut on his upper thigh. It was bleeding and his father could actually see that it was almost cut to the bone. He held a towel over the wound and performed Reiki while his wife called the ambulance. On arrival, the paramedics were surprised that the bleeding had stopped and said, "We don't know what you did to stop the bleeding but, whatever it was, you did a good job!" After receiving stitches and lots of Reiki from his Dad, James recovered quickly.

Part II

The Treatment

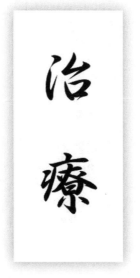

The Treatment Procedure

No matter how much discussion there is on the subject of Reiki treatments, the theory never quite matches up to the exquisiteness of the experience. Many regular clients claim they actually forget what a Reiki treatment feels like until that moment when they lie down and the practitioner places her hands on the body. At this point the memory of deep connection floods back and the client thankfully gives over to it.

If this is your first treatment you may be tempted to hold back in order to watch and wait. Once you feel comfortable in your environment and with your practitioner, try to loosen up to truly experience the full scope of a Reiki treatment.

On entering the clinic, your Reiki practitioner welcomes you and makes you comfortable. She may offer you a simple beverage, like green tea or water, as she talks to you briefly about Reiki; what it is, how it works, Reiki and contraindications, the benefits of Reiki, and possible responses during and after the treatment. You fill in a client record form together and she may ask you to sign a disclaimer.

Your practitioner asks if there is anything specific that you wish to work on and if you have any questions. Although a practitioner does not diagnose and Reiki works on the whole of the being, it is beneficial to be aware of a client's needs and expectations prior to a treatment. A practitioner is also naturally obligated to respect the client's confidence.

If necessary, the practitioner may add to the client record form that she has received consent from you for any extra practices or techniques you have discussed. Anything not considered to be a basic Reiki treatment is included in these notes.

After having carefully followed the conversation, the practitioner shares with you her treatment plan; explaining what she intends to do throughout the treatment. As Reiki is an intuitive practice this plan is subject to change, depending on the practitioner's energetic experiences during the treatment.

The practitioner asks you to lie down on your back on the treatment table. You are fully clothed, however the practitioner may suggest, for hygienic reasons and comfort, that you remove your shoes. A pillow may be placed under your head and under your knees to take the pressure off your lower back and a light blanket provided to help balance out your body temperature.

The first treatment that a client receives is often a general treatment which begins at the head and moves down through the front torso and limbs, then down the back torso and legs, finishing at the feet. The practitioner's hands do not physically touch private parts of the body, they are instead placed above the body at any sensitive points. There are many variations on this basic format with some treatments only covering the front of the body or not including limbs. It may also take anything from 45 minutes to an hour or more, depending on the length of your appointment time. A practitioner does not speak to you unnecessarily during a treatment as it may distract you from making that rare connection deep within yourself which supports healing and spiritual growth.

After the treatment, the practitioner allows you to rest for a short while before helping you to sit up. To support your body's clearing process you receive a glass of water. Together you discuss your experiences and decide whether follow-up treatments are required or not.

The practitioner offers follow-up support by giving you the opportunity to call or email if you find the cleansing process difficult or if you have further questions. A practitioner may also offer further information regarding how to learn to practice Reiki for yourself, emphasizing that the system of Reiki focuses on self-healing. You are also required to pay the practitioner at the end of the session.

LENGTH OF A TREATMENT

A Reiki treatment can, in reality, last from five minutes to an hour or even longer.

You may be offered a brief five-minute Reiki treatment by someone at work, or at a party, if you are unwell or have had an accident. It will not be possible, however, to book in for a five-minute treatment with a professional Reiki practitioner at a clinic.

As mentioned previously a professional Reiki treatment takes from 45 minutes up to an hour in length; with a longer session not always representing a more effective treatment.

Your body, in drawing on energy during a treatment, works like a sponge. It soaks up what it needs. Once it is "full" the body changes its focus from drawing energy to processing energy. After this has occurred the body can then begin to draw again. This is a simplistic perspective on the apparent workings of a Reiki treatment. Remember that you are already energy, as is the practitioner, and in life energy is constantly moving and merging.

Your practitioner can actually feel the rhythm of the energy being drawn and, sometimes, so can the client. It is possible for your practitioner to perceive a wide variety of sensations through his hands or body. He generally stays with his hands at one position on the body until the sensation diminishes or disappears altogether. This is an indication that energy is no longer being drawn and it is time for him to move to the following hand placement. For this reason it is difficult to regulate the timing of a Reiki treatment as the practitioner is relying on what is occurring energetically to dictate the timing of his hands' positions. The more experienced the practitioner, the easier this becomes.

According to the system of Reiki, professional Reiki practitioners should also be knowledgeable at working with Reiki on themselves. There is a constant striving on the practitioner's behalf to become a clearer pathway for the energy to move through. The less obstacles in the practitioner's energetic path, the easier it is for the client to draw more energy for healing.

It is important that a practitioner keeps the timing of a Reiki session accurate. This is a sure sign of professionalism and respect for his clients when he does not leave them sitting in the waiting room for too long, nor make them late for their own appointments.

Be Open to Healing

Humans are always connecting and disconnecting energetically from one another. Your healing can begin the moment you enter the clinic door. At this point the practitioner is already opening himself up to you, allowing the energy to flow. He is concentrating on you and tapping intuitively in to how he can support your self-healing process during the treatment. Be aware that your treatment has already begun and be open to begin to heal.

The entire ritualization of a Reiki session supports you in your healing: the clinic environment, the music, the hand positions, the practitioner's attitude and confidence and the length of the treatment. Together these elements come together to help make your Reiki session an entire experience that you can utilize to create change in your life.

INFORMATION YOUR PRACTITIONER NEEDS

When arriving at your Reiki treatment the Reiki practitioner asks you to fill in a client record form. Although Reiki is not diagnostic and does not offer a specific outcome or cure, a practitioner must equip herself with enough information to be able to treat her client professionally and knowledgeably.

Before, during and after a session, good two-way communication between you and your practitioner is essential. The greater the communication, the more effective the treatment. This does not infer that you are required to discuss your private life with a practitioner you do not know. It is about feeling confident enough in your environment to inform the practitioner of your needs and expectations. A Reiki session is not a counseling session nor is it a psychic reading.

Oh, My Back

Bernard was excited at the prospect of his first Reiki treatment. Bernard, however, did not tell his practitioner that he had a specific problem: lower back pain. He hid his pain, even as he climbed onto the table. The practitioner had asked him why he was there and if there was anything specific that he wanted to work on but Bernard said nothing – he wanted to see if the practitioner could spot his problem. This particular practitioner only worked down the front of her clients' bodies on their first treatment, spending a lot of time initially at the head. Bernard was irritated when he realized that the treatment was over and the practitioner had not even gone near his lower back pain. The practitioner should have made it clear to Bernard where she was planning to treat him and Bernard should not have been playing a game of hide and seek with his health and the practitioner. This was a case of a lack of clear communication between both the client and the practitioner.

Also required for the client record form is your name and contact details, a list of any medications that you are taking, the reason/s for your visit and anything else that you and your practitioner feel is relevant to the treatment. This form is completed in accordance with the practitioner's codes of ethics and practice, local and governmental laws, and privacy laws and is stored responsibly and securely.

In some countries, clients may access their client record forms to share with other health care workers to ensure that there is an across the board understanding of the client's wellbeing. If you wish the practitioner to fully comprehend your past history and current needs, you may like to bring notes from a previous health care worker. Be aware that Reiki practitioners have a varying knowledge of other therapies and conventional western medicine. If you are still in consultation with other health care workers your Reiki practitioner may recommend that you inform them that you are also attending a Reiki treatment.

Client Records

... for professional indemnity insurance purposes, it is important to keep proper records of consultations, treatment and advice. Client records comprise files, notes of treatment, prescriptions, medical history, personal details, letters to other practitioners, test results, x-rays, diagnosis, family history, photographs and correspondence with clients.

Complementary Medicine: Ethics and Law
Michael Weir

Although a Reiki practitioner may not require as detailed client records as a Naturopath for example, the practitioner still needs to be aware of your basic medical history. Your client record form also includes details as to what you and your practitioner discussed prior to, during and after the treatment and your practitioner's recommendations including the booking of future treatments, if any.

A practitioner may also request that you sign a disclaimer. Many of these are standard and re-iterate your awareness of what is included in your treatment. The disclaimer also acknowledges that a Reiki treatment is not diagnostic in nature, but always read it carefully before signing.

Reiki and Your Privacy

Privacy laws exist to protect your personal information.

According to Michael Weir, author of *Complementary Medicine: Ethics and Law*, personal information represents information that can identify an individual. Information that does not allow a particular person to be identified is not covered by privacy laws.

Health Information is Personal Information:

- *About a person's individual health or disability at any time ie past, current or future.*
- *About expressed wishes regarding future health services.*
- *About health services provided to a person.*
- *Collected while providing the health service.*
- *Health information can include medical information, name, address, Medicare number, notes or opinions about a person's health status.*

Complementary Medicine: Ethics and Law
Michael Weir

A Reiki practitioner is obliged to respect a client's confidentiality. Your practitioner should be considerate of your needs when asking questions including what is asked, how and where.

None of His Business

Claire, 26, was visiting a Reiki practitioner for the first time. She was dealing with mild depression and stress. When her male practitioner asked her why she wanted a treatment she explained briefly how she was feeling and the reason for her visit. The practitioner began to ask her questions; for example, was she on medication or currently seeing a doctor? Her practitioner then went on to ask her how many times a week she had sex. Claire felt suddenly intimidated and wanted to leave the room.

As a Reiki treatment is not diagnostic, and has no contraindications, information requested by the practitioner should be basic and germane to the Reiki treatment. If you feel that the questions are too personal or irrelevant to the treatment at hand you have every right to refuse to answer them.

If you feel that your privacy has not been respected, boundaries have been crossed, or your practitioner has breached his duty of confidence, then you should immediately contact the relevant authority. Depending on the severity of the issue you may wish to contact the practitioner's Reiki association, national industry body or the police department.

The "Too Pushy" Practitioner

Rod was recovering from prostate cancer. His daughter bought him a Reiki treatment gift voucher as a present. The practitioner was professional and caring and Rod really enjoyed the treatment. She told him that she would call him in three days time to check that he was dealing well with the treatment, which she did. Rod explained that he was feeling healthy and thanked her for her solicitousness, which he personally felt was over and above the call of duty of a practitioner. A week later the practitioner rang again, and she continued to call every week over the next month to check on Rod's health. She finished each call with the same question, asking if he felt another Reiki treatment might be beneficial. Eventually Rod stopped answering the phone, asking his wife to take it in case it was "that Reiki practitioner" again. Rod didn't want to insult her but he felt that his privacy was being intruded upon.

Each clinic should hold a privacy policy that can be made available on request. This policy reassures you that your personal details are appropriately stored and that they will not be shared or sold on to others.

THE SAFETY OF REIKI

Reiki is a safe practice. This is due to the fact that a Reiki practitioner does not manipulate or diagnose nor prescribe medication.

The Reiki practitioner learns techniques that support her in strengthening her energetic connection to the universal life force energy while also building her inner ability to hold that energy. The practitioner offers that energy to the client who, at a largely unconscious level, draws on this energy, taking it to where it is needed most. You, the client, control the situation energetically by your own needs and your unique relationship to the Reiki treatment.

This simple explanation is the accepted viewpoint of most Reiki practitioners. Clients also readily accept this simple, yet enigmatic, description of how a practitioner and client relate energetically in a Reiki context. Although this is the case, a number of myths concerning Reiki's safety have managed to ingratiate themselves into the Reiki world. These myths all have commonsense answers, the client just needs to be able to think straight for a moment to realize this. Following are three common Reiki myths.

1. Do not perform Reiki on a person with a pacemaker as it may stop the pacemaker from working.

Commonsense Answer: Reiki is a very subtle energy that works toward creating balance in the body. It *does not* affect the running of electrical appliances and a pacemaker is an electrical appliance. According to this myth, Reiki practitioners should be careful when performing Reiki around electrical equipment which, consequently, would result in a Reiki practitioner being unable to use a walkman or iPod when working with Reiki. There is no documented evidence of Reiki practitioners affecting their music players or any other electrical equipment.

2. Do not perform Reiki on broken bones before a doctor sets them as they may set incorrectly.

Commonsense Answer: Reiki is a very subtle energy that works toward creating balance in the body, therefore, the client with the broken bone may experience less swelling and pain and may feel calmer. If it were an everyday possibility for Reiki practitioners to mend bones in a couple of minutes, as is suggested by this myth, there would be some very exciting documented evidence of these miracle healings, while, unfortunately, there are none.

3. Do not use Reiki on a client who is under anesthetic as she may wake up during surgery.

Commonsense Answer: There is no documented evidence of this occurring during surgery. Reiki is a very subtle energy that works toward creating balance, therefore many aspects of the operating room procedure may be supported by offering Reiki during an operation. It is possible that there is a calmer and more grounded quality in the operating room, a greater clarity of mind for the doctors and nurses and that the patient can draw energy to where she most needs it at the time. For your peace of mind also remember that anesthesiologists constantly monitor the health of their patients throughout surgery and will always adjust the anesthetic accordingly.

Such myths abound due to a serious lack of experiential understanding of Reiki on the behalf of the practitioner who suggested the myths in the first place. The practitioner may feel uncertain about the extent of her ability and create rules (or accept the rules of others) to falsely steady her Reiki hands and the honesty in her eyes. A wad of rules supports a practitioner's bravado; yet the confidence gained from creating such myths is temporary and ultimately misleading. Rules create fear in the client and practitioner and that is not, and must never be, a part of the system of Reiki. This is a good reason why all Reiki practitioners should come from a place of self-reflection and Reiki experience in order to quell the desire for power over others.

Although Reiki is safe, there are inherent risks in any therapeutic situation and this relates to a practitioner's duty of care to the client. To support this professional role it is often recommended that a practitioner has a basic knowledge of anatomy and physiology, recognize emergency and First Aid situations, and understands Occupational Health and Safety, privacy laws and ethics in relation to her practice.

Your Physical Position

During your Reiki treatment, the most common scenario entails you lying on a treatment table. A Reiki treatment table is the same as a massage table but it does not need extra padding or require extra strengthening, which might be the case if you were to receive a deep tissue massage.

Reiki treatments may also be performed on a futon on the floor, shiatsu style, but this depends upon your practitioner's dexterity.

If you are unable to comfortably lie on a table, which might be the case if you are heavily pregnant for example, or if you have acute back pain then you can discuss with your practitioner what the best position for you might be. This could simply be on a chair or seated, or propped up, on the floor.

If you stand throughout a treatment, which is also possible, it needs to be taken into account that the energy may relax you to the point that you slowly begin to sway. Standing may not allow you to fully relax into the energy.

Your position does not affect the efficacy of your Reiki treatment – if you are uncomfortable however, you may be less open to healing.

What to Wear for your Reiki Treatment

- Comfortable clothes for lying on a treatment table.
- Removable belt.
- Loose, or no, tie.
- Limited jewelry, as it may get in the practitioner's way.
- You may prefer to remove your watch for comfort.
- Easy shoes to slip on/off.
- Clean socks.
- Don't forget to turn off your cell/mobile phone.

Reiki practitioners can be also be found in hospitals today, largely as volunteers – though this is gradually changing as more people see the benefits that Reiki can bring to the hospital environment. Some hospital policies accept Reiki practitioners in the operating room, if so requested by the patient. Julie Motz's book, *Hands of Life*, discusses her work with Dr Mehmet Oz, where she performed Reiki with his transplant patients before, during and after surgery. A hospital environment is unique and, depending upon the situation, the Reiki practitioner needs to be aware of any procedures or emergencies taking place. He needs to work around medical equipment and other health care workers – and yet his presence can be of great service to everyone in this setting. Flexibility on the practitioner's behalf is very important. Sometimes just holding a client's hand with the intent that the client takes whatever he needs at that moment in his life is all that is required and can, in itself, be enormously beneficial.

Being There with Reiki

In a tea producing village in the Indian Himalaya, two western Reiki practitioners traipsed from house to house offering free Reiki treatments. The local school teacher, who hoped to bring some healing to her local community, guided them. They entered a small wooden house where in the tiny front room the two practitioners slid in beside a bed where a skinny old man lay motionless and asleep. The teacher told them he was dying. Not wanting to intrude upon this man's privacy, they simply held his hands, sitting with him quietly. He lay apparently unaware throughout. When it was time for the practitioners to leave they shuffled back out of the room. Glancing back through the doorway, they watched the old man lift his head from his pillow with effort and waveringly place his hands together in the namaste position. He then raised them to his forehead as a sign of gratitude and sank back into his bed. "Namaste" the practitioners murmured together and raised their own clasped hands to their foreheads in response, offering thanks for the teaching.

HAND POSITIONS AND SPECIFIC ILLNESSES

Hands-on healing itself was very popular at that beginning of the 20th century in Japan with teachers like Eguchi Toshihiro reportedly having more than 500,000 students. He would teach tenohira (hands-on healing) in halls with hundreds of students present. On the other hand, the founder of Reiki, Usui Mikao, had his dôjô (teaching place) in Aoyama, Tôkyô and then Nakano Ku and students would come there to learn about healing and spirituality on a likely much less grand scale. It is thought that the system of Reiki may, initially, have never used hand positions at all, with students simply being asked to set their intent to draw on the energy of their teacher, Usui Mikao. He was an energetic master and it is questionable that Reiki teachers today have the ability to emulate this practice. Hand positions are taught to practitioners to offer them tools (their hands) to help direct their thoughts and intent. During the latter years of Usui Mikao's life he taught a number of naval officers specific hand positions to support them on their naval vessels.

One of these was a surgeon called Hayashi Chûjirô. It is thought that Usui Mikao had relied upon Hayashi's medical knowledge to develop a system where hands were placed upon specific positions on the body for various illnesses. A manual exists from the original naval officers' society which lists these positions. In the 1930s, Hayashi Chûjirô used a very similar manual in his own practice.

Hayashi Chûjirô's manual allowed him to bring together a medical framework with an energetic practice. Although Reiki supports the body in taking energy to where it is needed, perhaps a more structured or technical system was appealing to the naval officers. The positions in the manuals reflected a basic commonsense understanding of where it might be reasonable to place hands depending upon the client's illness. Beginners, with little experience, might also find such a manual beneficial rather than relying on their underdeveloped intuition.

Commonsense and intuition are the main factors that a professional Reiki practitioner utilizes when deciding where to place her hands today. There is little commonsense in placing hands on someone's big toe when it is the ear that is hurting. Naturally, a practitioner places hands as close to the area of interest as possible. Although this is the case it is still up to the body to draw the energy wherever it is needed. But how, then, do you treat emotional issues or more general health issues?

A 45-minute Reiki treatment includes the practitioner covering the head and major organs of the body with her hands. Limbs may also be treated. This is a general Reiki treatment which also takes into account any illness or issue that a client presents.

A practitioner also senses intuitively, and even physically, where to place the hands and how long they should remain in position. A practitioner who works in this manner is more likely to be effective than one who works solely from a book; she listens to the body and responds accordingly.

Hands do not need to be placed directly on the affected area. When Usui Mikao began teaching hands-on healing, he apparently asked practitioners to place their hands at positions on the head only. The head plays an important role in the functioning of all bodily systems. Afterwards, the hands would be placed on the body, directed by intuition only.

Let Reiki do the Healing

After Jenny studied Reiki, she enthusiastically began to offer treatments to her friends and family. Jenny's dad had recently dislocated his knee and was having trouble getting around – she thought he would be a perfect candidate. He was unsure about "this Reiki thing" but said he would have a go. Jenny sat next to his chair, asked him to relax and placed both hands on his troubled knee. She did this for about half an hour once a day, for three consecutive days. At the end of the three sessions she asked her dad if there was any improvement in his knee. He disappointingly shook his head and then remarked, "But I can sure hear better now."

Hands-on or Hands-off the Body

Reiki practitioners are generally encouraged to touch during a Reiki treatment by placing their loosely cupped hands onto the body, molding them to the client's physical form. The main reason for this is that touch is one of humanity's major senses and, as such, is integral to optimal human performance. Touch reminds you that life is a human experience; with it you can feel yourself and others, experiencing a physical connection to the world around you. Touch is a pleasure, and the more humanity touches and is touched, the more stimulated, motivated and active life becomes.

Touch is often not encouraged in contemporary society due to laws that aim to protect the individual. Though certainly created for societal benefit, the associated advantages of safe touching are consequently ignored. In the first instance, a Reiki treatment can relieve a great deal of stress and anxiety by simply allowing the client the chance to accept touch in a non-manipulative or threatening manner, without any sexual implications.

History of Modern Touch

From the beginning, Freud and other psychoanalysts established a no-touch rule in the therapeutic relationship, even though touch had long been considered an important healing tool. (Durana, 1998). Using touch was considered to have a detrimental effect on transference and countertransference, as well as confuse ego boundaries for both the client and therapist (Gutheil & Gabbard, 1993). However, this stance ignores the value of touch as a powerful therapeutic tool and excludes a whole range of body-centered approaches that can facilitate growth.

The Use of Reiki in Psychotherapy
Mary Ann LaTorre

Reiki treatments are not necessarily skin touching skin. It is irrelevant to the Reiki practitioner whether he touches the skin or clothing while offering the treatment. The only items of clothing that may be required to be removed for a Reiki treatment are a coat and shoes.

The Science behind Healing through Touch or Near-Touch

A variety of electrical, electronic, magnetic and other energetic phenomena take place within healthy tissue as a consequence of the communications needed to coordinate cellular activities. The resulting energy fields are radiated from the hands of the healthy individual. Whether caused by physical or emotional trauma, 'the wound that does not heal' is a wound that is not receiving the natural regulatory signals needed to initiate and coordinate repair processes. When healthy tissue is brought close to such a wound, essential information is transferred via the energy field, communication channels open and the healing process is 'jump started'.

Energy Medicine: The Scientific Basis
James L. Oschman

Reiki is safe touch, something many clients crave. Once this craving is satisfied then the human body can open up to allow healing at a very deep level. Safe touch is the key that opens the door, it promises your spirit that you are protected from harm, allowing you to heal.

A Reiki practitioner does not touch any private parts of the body and may ask you prior to your treatment if there are any other areas of your body where you may not feel comfortable receiving physical touch. Consequently, these body parts are not touched, but, if appropriate, he may place his hands just off your body with the same intent and focus as if his hands were placed directly on the body.

Private parts of the body refer to a woman's breasts and pelvic region and may also refer to her buttocks. For men the groin area and sometimes the buttocks are considered off limits. Reiki practitioners need to be aware of a client's personal and cultural boundaries to ensure that the client feels relaxed, calm and, most importantly, safe.

A practitioner must not put his hands directly on burns or any areas that are too painful to touch. In case of infection a practitioner may also be required to wear gloves and in a hospital situation wear clothing that protects the client and/or the practitioner. None of these circumstances should affect the quality of the Reiki that the practitioner offers to the client.

REIKI AND NEGATIVE ENERGY

Reiki is the energy of everything and is often described as universal life force energy. Within universal energy there is both negative and positive energy. In Japan, these two elements are called In and Yo and are more commonly known in the West by their Chinese names of Yin and Yang.

In and Yo are not words for *bad* and *good* but rather representations of dual elements – the flipsides of a coin. In and Yo also represent other dualities such as Earth and Heaven, female and male, the moon and sun. By balancing and blending dual elements within yourself you create a non-dual existence, one where you begin to resonate fully with universal energy.

Life is not Black and White

The wise understand that clarity and darkness do not have separate natures; their true natures are nondualistic. Deluded people make absolute distinctions between good and evil, between a good path and a bad path, between black and white, while those who are wise clearly understand that these pairs do not have separate natures. The true nature of all things is nondualistic.

Describing the Indescribable
Master Hsing Yun

To minimize this sense of duality, try replacing the terms positive and negative energy with two other opposites, such as Earth and Heaven energy. For example, too much Earth energy can create a stuck feeling where you feel you cannot escape or move. Too much Heavenly energy, on the other hand, might mean that you are "off with the fairies" or that your "head is in the clouds". Neither of these energies is innately bad but both, if untended, reflect an unbalanced state that can create problems within your life. Balance them out, allow the clouds to draw you out of your stuck environment and allow the ground to keep you moving ahead clearly and purposefully with each step.

This is what a Reiki treatment can do for you. It is not about taking the negative away and filling yourself up with positive energy. True healing takes place as the two forces balance out harmoniously. To heal, you eventually need to face all sides of yourself including your fears and darkest issues. A Reiki treatment can bring these issues to the surface and offer you the opportunity to take responsibility for your personal spiritual progress, letting go of self-condemnation and working toward balance instead.

Believing that you are taking on "negative" energy from another is a reflection of your own lack of inner balance. By working toward complete balance you begin to overcome fears and insecurities which are the breeding ground for the creation of dualistic concepts such as good and bad.

Take this responsibility into your own hands, own it and live life in acceptance. Move away from the need to label your experiences as good, bad, positive or negative. Labeling things restricts their energetic flow and restricts *your* energetic flow. Allow your eyes to be opened and not shuttered by the use of labels. Move instead into a state of union with the universe; it is there that your obstacles have the opportunity to resolve. This in turn will produce healing and long lasting peace of mind.

YOUR INTENT

Your Reiki practitioner has explained that the success of the Reiki treatment is not only in his hands (so to speak), it also depends upon you; your ability to be open and relaxed and willing to heal. You remember your maxim, "I am open to receive whatever it is that I may need at this exact moment in my life." Your body listens and responds allowing Reiki to seep below the everyday shell of protection that you have created around yourself.

A realization is enforced within you that the practitioner can *do* very little to you, only you can heal yourself. Even if the practitioner tried to make something happen – if you didn't want it, then it wouldn't happen.

Setting your thoughts, your intent, to allow self-healing to occur is a powerful affirmation. It reminds you of your personal power and that the practitioner is there merely to support you in that process. The more lucid your understanding of this principle, the deeper the healing.

The Importance of Intent

I said that the cure itself is a certain leaf, but in addition to the drug there is a certain charm, which if someone chants when he makes use of it, the medicine altogether restores him to health, but without the charm there is no profit from the leaf.

Plato (Charmides, 155-6)

Intent is powerful. The way you view your health and healing affects how effectively you heal. Many people today take medication, in swallowing a pill they open themselves to the healing that it may offer them. It is not just the content of the pill that heals, there are more factors at play here. Most important is the role of the placebo effect.

A placebo is inert, a non-treatment – it is not meant to do anything. At the same time it is also accepted that between 30% to 60% of patients receiving placebos respond to them.[23] Placebos may be inert (a sugar pill for example) but their effect can be meaningful to the user and therefore affect the user. Daniel E. Moerman and Dr. Wayne B. Jonas call this the "meaning response". Humans take meaning from everything they see and experience and respond to it, in reality there is no such thing as a "non-treatment".[24]

Moerman and Jonas relate two studies on coronary surgery (the binding of the bilateral internal mammary arteries as a treatment for angina pectoris) where patients receiving sham surgery did as well – with 80% of patients substantially improving – as those receiving the active procedure. In another study, users taking branded aspirin found that it worked better than the same product which was non-branded.[25] The power of the human mind cannot be underestimated.

Moerman and Jonas also discuss the ritual around healing that adds meaning to the doctor/patient experience; the doctor's white coat, blood and the therapeutic quality of the doctor's manner. All of these aspects add a meaningful response to the patient's healing experience.

The cyclical nature of life is reflected in your own healing. The clearer your intent to heal, the greater the healing and, consequently, the easier it is to set your intent to continue that healing.

Clarity of Intent = Improved Self-Healing

The clarity of pure consciousness cannot be perceived until all impure intentions have been removed from it.

Describing the Indescribable
Master Hsing Yun

You lie on the treatment table in the professional environment of the clinic and the friendly and encouraging practitioner assures you that you can create change in your life and that self-healing is in your hands. Your confidence (or growing confidence) in this ritual is what opens you up to allow the healing to occur. Reiki treatments are rituals. The stronger the connection that you make to the ritual, the easier it becomes for you to unlock your healing ability. Don't dwell upon it, just let it flow through you and, soon, you will reach the home of inner quietude.

ENERGY CENTERS AND YOUR TREATMENT

The system of Reiki is an energetic system and therefore has at its base a concept of how energy works. Depending upon which culture a teaching is based upon, this energetic concept will vary.

As the system of Reiki is a Japanese practice from the early 1900s, it is relevant to look at the energetic concept which lay at the base of Japanese culture at that time. Many martial arts and Ki practices were formalized in Japan in the early 1900s including karate, judo and aikidô and they considered the hara or tanden to be the center of the body's energetic powerhouse.

The word hara literally means stomach, abdomen or belly in Japanese. Energy is stored at this point from where it expands throughout the whole body.

Usui Mikao's teachings focus on building energy in the hara. The self-practice techniques which have been passed down from the early 1900s work at strengthening the hara. From Hawayo Takata's diary notes it can be seen that she, too, was taught to practice in this manner, though she did not appear to overtly teach it in her classes. Once the system of Reiki became more westernized the chakra system (an energetic system from India that has been incorporated into the New Age movement) was introduced and is now commonly used in the West.

In traditional Japanese teachings and exercises today the hara system is still the main focus for building a person's energy.

As a client it is not necessary for you to focus on any energy centers, this can undermine the strength of your intent. Reiki practitioners in the past have been known to unwisely make comments about a client's chakras. For example, the statement, "I opened up your heart chakra but your throat is still blocked" is the result of a lack of professionalism and experience on the practitioner's behalf. Words like "open", "blocked" and "closed" can cause damage to a client's self worth and are extremely unempowering. The client may be unaware that all energetic interpretation is subjective. Such methods of practice do not support long-term healing but exist only to build a practitioner's ego.

From an energetic perspective such a statement is also false. Whichever energetic concept a practitioner may base her understanding of Reiki on, universal truths still apply. All energetic centers within the body connect and are interrelated, as individual parts of the human system do not work in isolation.

Some practitioners might work with chakras while others work with the hara, others again might not work with any kind of energetic concept at all. Other ways to understand the movement of energy in the body exist in various cultures or therapies with some of them talking about reflexology points, shiatsu points, acupuncture points and meridians.

All that matters at the end of the session is how you feel and that in the long run you begin to feel healthier, happier and more connected to life.

Your Practitioner's Choice

Remember that each practitioner's energetic understanding is unique. The sensing of energy and energy centers in or around the body is subjective. A practitioner's interpretation of where your energy centers are will depend upon her cultural and experiential understanding as well as her Reiki training and her personal choice of language.

YOUR TREATMENT AND REIKI ATTUNEMENTS

Some clients are unsure what the difference is between receiving a Reiki treatment or, during a Reiki course, receiving an attunement as both support your healing process. Research indicates that when Usui Mikao began teaching there may have been no difference between a treatment and attunements. Reiju, the Japanese word for the early form of attunement, is an energetic ritual connecting the teacher and student. Literally translated, reiju means *spiritual blessing*.

Initially, Usui Mikao used reiju to create an energetic space to support the student in drawing whatever energy the student required at that moment in time. There were no true clients during this period, as all clients became students of Usui Mikao – though it is likely that not all progressed to the status of deshi, a formal student. Whoever came for reiju would likely receive practices for self-healing that were to be continued at home, such as meditations.

In time this changed and, according to Usui Mikao's memorial stone, he became known as a healer and many people would visit him for hands-on healing. Hands-on healing was very popular in Japan at that time. This was just one aspect of his teachings and perhaps the hands-on healing was a development toward a more physical, ritualized practice which he felt was more accessible and, in the short-term, more supportive of his clients.

There are two major differences between receiving a Reiki treatment and receiving an attunement or reiju, with the first being the intent and the second, the procedure.

There are many layers to intent. There is conscious intent such as the Reiki maxim, and then there are many layered unconscious understandings beneath that. During a Reiki session these might include a practitioner's unconscious intent that a treatment shall take a specific amount of time to perform and that it shall occur in a certain manner. The practitioner also expects the actions of this treatment to be effective in the context of a Reiki treatment.

Part of the, often unconscious, intent behind an attunement or reiju performed by a teacher is in the context of ongoing self-healing work for the student. The attunement or reiju is the initiator

of a continuing energetic connection and development
teacher and student with the expectation that the stu
with self-healing at home.

The Reiki treatment procedure is an extended ritual where the hands are tools that support the practitioner and client in connecting to the ritual of healing. The practitioner's set-up is more ritualistic and physical and this ritual is integral to the meaningful aspect of the healing process when receiving a treatment.

An attunement or reiju has less ritual and therefore requires more experience on the teacher's behalf to be highly effective. There is less for a teacher to be able to use, or to connect with, to create the space for the student to draw the energy through.

Stimulating your Body's Natural Healing Process (Internal Economy)

Perhaps only when a friend, relative, or healer indicates some level of social support (for example, by performing a ritual) is the individual's internal economy able to act.[26]

Deconstructing the Placebo Effect and Finding the Meaning Response
Daniel E. Moerman, PhD, and Wayne B. Jonas, MD

Both treatments and attunements or reiju are effective methods for clearing energy in the body as you work toward re-balancing the body. Receiving reiju or an attunement does not, however, make you a Level I Reiki student. For that you must complete an entire course with a teacher where you learn the Reiki meditations, techniques and history and gain a clearer understanding of what Reiki is.

Sensing Reiki

Winds of Desire

//

As a boat on the water is swept away by strong wind and thrown off course, even one of the senses on which the mind focuses can carry away one's intelligence.

//

Bhagavad Gita: Chaper 2, Verse 67

The human senses are sight, touch, hearing, smell and taste. A sixth sense is often called intuition and in *Your Reiki Treatment* it is referred to as the spiritual sense. These senses help humanity learn about, and navigate, the world. In the past, those with highly developed senses were often dubbed as mystics and yet, humanity constantly uses these senses in daily life. Senses are the human antennae and as you grow up you begin to intellectually understand what it is to use them and what their benefits are.

To cross a road you use your ears to listen out for traffic, your sight to see the oncoming cars and the path you are about to walk, your touch to move easily from the footpath onto the road, perhaps your smell to check that everything is safe.

You are born with a natural ability to use one or more of your senses more than another and at the same time you also hone separate senses depending on your life choices. Some of your senses are more responsive than others depending on how you use them. If you are a cook then perhaps your sense of smell and taste is very sharp. If you are a sculptor your sense of touch, your spiritual awareness and perhaps sight, might earn you your living. A data analyst uses her sense of sight to read (or ears to hear an audio tape), sense of touch to use a computer and taste to slurp endless cups of coffee.

At the base of these senses, which all Reiki practitioners and clients experience during a Reiki treatment (though may not all feel), is energy. Energy is expressed through our six senses.

When you begin to consciously experience sensations with Reiki you may not know what it is meant to feel like or how you should read it. No matter what age you are, the realization of an energetic experience may surprise you. This realization ensures that, although you may not be able to see Reiki, there is no denying that you are still drawing what you require during your Reiki treatment. As the Reiki moves through you, your senses become clearer and more acute. Do not muddy them with human interpretation.

Sensing without Attachment

//

The ancients used to say, "When no thought arises, the whole world is clear. When the six senses move, the world is covered with clouds."

//

Describing the Indescribable
Master Hsing Yun

Your responses are not the point of your treatment. Know that you are receiving a Reiki treatment, your senses are open to take their healing journey and your practitioner has made herself available to support you on that journey.

Some people may claim to sense and understand a great deal from a Reiki treatment. It is possible that this person is energetically advanced – if this is the case then the person will not be attached to the sensations. There is also the possibility that the person is so weak that she is being tossed to and fro by all that she senses around her. She is unable to control her sensitivity and is attached to the desire to "know" intangible things. This person is in a state of imbalance and needs to develop a stronger inner self and energetic understanding before treating others.

SENSING REIKI VISUALLY

A Reiki treatment can surprise clients when they see bright colors or specific images for no apparent reason. This is a common Reiki phenomenon, though not one experienced by everyone.

Imagine that you are enjoying a wonderfully relaxing Reiki treatment; you are almost dozing off in a beautiful twilight space of awareness when suddenly the sky lights up and you are enjoying the most amazing fireworks – with your eyes closed. You are still very relaxed and unconcerned and only if you are lucky do you remember afterwards what happened during the treatment.

Yes, it can mean a number of things. Some metaphysicians state that a certain color indicates a specific state of mind, activity in an energy center, or they may even use the colors to decide upon the state of a client's spiritual development. Some of these conclusions may well be interesting and in some cases true and yet no-one can guarantee that they are correct. Red may well indicate passion, but it could also symbolize anger. Cultural consequences can also affect one's interpretation with red representing good luck in some Asian countries. Who decides which of these is the correct energetic translation?

The conceptual String Theory gives a glimpse of how little humanity may understand about its experience. It states that space is filled with vibrating strings. These strings create the four dimensions of height, width, depth and time, plus an additional seven dimensions which cannot be perceived.

Your Limited Vantage Point

We don't see them because of the way we see...like an ant walking along a lily pad...we could be floating within a grand, expansive, higher-dimensional space.

The Fabric of the Cosmos
Brian Greene

It is possible that limited perceptive abilities restrict a true under-standing of what these visions may mean. Judgments formed about the results of sense stimulation are in fact attachment to the senses. Both the client and practitioner can become fixated on the idea that colors are a significant part of the treatment. When a practitioner becomes attached to this limited perspective, he needs to have the same outcome at every treatment as a personal validation of his ability. The client, too, may want to repeat the same experience be-cause without it the Reiki treatment may appear to be ineffective. These misunderstandings lead both the practitioner and client away from the profundity of the Reiki experience. There is so much more to life than is rationally understood and by labeling things from a limited perception, only limited healing can occur.

But don't be misled into thinking that colors are unimportant. When you are lying on the massage table and those colors begin to move and snake their way around your inner world, the uni-verse is definitely speaking directly to you. It is saying, "Things are beginning to change in your life. Let go, and open up further to ex-perience this treatment, to let the energy flow freely. As a human you have been given the gift of the senses; these senses are indi-cating, by their flow and ebb, that your life, too, is changing and flowing. Be thankful, enjoy and let go." This understanding in itself might be the healing that you require.

SENSING REIKI PHYSICALLY

Western culture has been in denial regarding the link between the physical body and other aspects of our human condition for centuries. Up until recently it has believed that many illnesses can be treated with a pill without taking into consideration the relationship between the doctor and patient and other more abstract factors that appear to work hand-in-hand with the physical realm. The reason for this can possibly be traced back to a major event in the 17th century:

The Origins of the Mind-Body Disconnection

...Rene Descartes, the philosopher and founding father of modern medicine, was forced to make a turf deal with the Pope in order to get the human bodies he needed for dissection. Descartes agreed he wouldn't have anything to do with the soul, the mind, or the emotions – those aspects of human experience under the virtually exclusive jurisdiction of the church at the time – if he could claim the physical realm as his own.

Molecules of Emotion
Candace B. Pert, Ph.D.

This may account for therapies such as the system of Reiki being required to prove themselves inline with modern western medical structures and methods, even if the structures in place are inadequate in measuring the subjective experience of Reiki.

During a Reiki treatment, you may sense things physically occurring in and around your body. You may begin to shake, tremble, suffer sharp needle-like pains, experience palpitations or sweating. You may feel as if there are many hands offering you Reiki. It may become difficult to take deep breaths or you suddenly feel so cold that you require a blanket. You might even snore or hum while receiving a treatment. These physical sensations may not all sound pleasant but as you undergo them you are generally far from concerned. It is as if the body needs to respond but you are mentally and emotionally fine. There is an anchor inside you that a Reiki treatment touches; someplace immovable and true.

Did My Fingers Twitch?

Tina was curious about Reiki. Before her treatment she asked the practitioner what seemed like a zillion questions as to how it worked and what it would do to her. Her practitioner explained that she could not tell Tina exactly what might happen as it is a totally individual experience for each client; she may feel something or she may not. Either way, the practitioner assured her that the Reiki would still be working away at, and supporting, her healing process. As Tina's body began to relax into the treatment the practitioner noticed her fingers flexing, then her arms rising off the table, slowly and deliberately. Her hands began to touch her forehead gently, and then the center of her chest. Her fingers twirled and danced around her body. As the treatment came to a close Tina's arms and hands rested back in their place on the table as if nothing had happened. After the treatment, Tina sat up and looked at the practitioner and said 'Did my fingers twitch? I'm sure I felt them twitching!" She had been in such a connected and peaceful state, she was unaware of the beautiful dance-like movements she had been making for the last half hour.

You do not need to associate these physical sensations with any specific healing or meaning; a practitioner knows that the movement of energy in the body is at their cause. Physical movement occurs during a Reiki treatment because energy has a dynamic effect on the physical body.

SENSING REIKI AURALLY

Mystics and geniuses have claimed throughout history to sense voices, ethereal music, words or strange sounds. Robert Schumann believed he was taking dictation from Schubert's ghost, Abraham in the Old Testament believed that God instructed him to sacrifice his only son (but fortunately for the family was then instructed to stop and was given a sacrificial ram in his place), Charles Dickens claimed he was told dirty stories in church by one of his novel's characters making him laugh out loud.

It is as if the senses, when moved to new depths of understanding, can pick up things from other planes, perhaps timeless planes beyond the normality of daily existence.

Old Friends

At 55-years of age, Pamela began making some drastic changes to her life. To support this process she joined a Reiki course. During the Reiki treatment she received from her classmate, she heard a distinctive voice saying, "Hi, it's me. Tommy". Afterward, as she related this to the class, she remarked that she didn't know anyone called Tommy. As the students continued discussing their treatments, Pamela began to cry. Everyone quieted down as Pamela spoke up, "I remember. Tommy was my imaginary friend when I was a little girl."

What it meant, or who Tommy really was or is, is immaterial. This experience for Pamela was a treasured connection with her childhood that she needed to internally absorb rather than mentally understand. As is the way of these mystical experiences, it gave Pamela something to hold onto, to encourage her to continue working toward becoming whole.

Some Reiki clients talk of hearing a repetitive sound they believe is the heartbeat of the universe. This primordial connection with the inner rhythms of the planet and the universe is profound. Many clients come to realize that this sound has always vibrated through their bodies but they have been too distracted to hear or notice it. By taking the time for peace and quiet, and to soak in what feels like a Reiki bath, this universal pulse is conducted with more nuance. The rhythmic sounds may sometimes correlate to the sound you hear when you place your ear to a shell; the vast sound of a tidal ocean moving in and out on the sea breeze.

The marathon monks in Japan, who complete seven years of austerity training, become known as Living Buddhas. Only a handful of monks have completed this training and if they are unsuccessful they are expected to commit ritual suicide. At the end of their incredibly strenuous 1000-day practice their hyper-acuity is so pronounced that they can apparently hear ash falling from an incense stick. This ability arises from learning to live in unison with the movement of the universe.

Music, celestial in nature, has been known to move some clients emotionally during a Reiki treatment. The otherworldliness of these sounds, apparent to the client alone, brings an impression of angels singing. Its ethereal beauty draws them away from their everyday lives taking them to a heavenly realm surrounded by peace and love.

These other worlds of sound remind us that we are not just five senses and a baseball cap. Accept these encounters with the unknown and be thankful but do not try to manipulate them to fit into any fantasized scenario to make them reasonable or wise. Their wisdom lies in their presence alone.

SENSING REIKI WITH SMELL & TASTE

A smell sends a message to the brain which stimulates the hypothalamus to send out signals to the rest of the body. As a part of the emotional limbic system, the hypothalamus interprets smells as good, bad, pleasant or offensive. These communications tell you that you are hungry (because it smells SO good) or, in cases of unpleasant smells, these signals can suppress your hunger. All of our senses are interlinked; however, smell and taste commonly affect one another.

As you become more open to life and what exists within it, seen and unseen, you begin to experience sensations such as unusual smells and tastes that are related to your healing journey. For example, the previously mentioned marathon monks in Japan are said to be able to catch a whiff of meals being cooked miles away. This is due to their practice that supports them in becoming One with existence – they can even become One with the cook from the next village if that is their intent.

During a Reiki treatment you may smell something which reminds you of an event or period in your life. Smell may often link you to an emotional connection on a conscious level. Sometimes, the smell makes no sense whatsoever and you must accept it for what it is.

Occasionally there are also smells which you can relate to a specific issue. It is interesting to be aware of these smells. A smell is an unusual sign from the body letting you know that change is occurring. That in itself can be an affirming message.

Smelling Your Health

Claire smelt this terribly foul odor during her Reiki treatment. She wondered if it originated from her stomach as she had been experiencing indigestion problems After her treatment she had mild diarrhea for a couple of days and by the end of the week her indigestion had disappeared.

Commonsense told her the smell was due to her current physical shape – she had guessed what it related to. The diarrhea must have been the body emptying itself of something she no longer needed or that was not working well for her.

Other smells might be of flowers, incense or even cigarette smoke.

Old Habits

While performing the treatment, the practitioner briefly smelt cigarette smoke surrounding her and the client. After the treatment, the client reported that she had tasted a stale cigarette taste in her mouth – she had stopped smoking two years earlier.

As residue leaves your body, your new awareness actually alerts you to the process. Metallic tastes may also occur. These are often toxins leaving the body and may be the result of an excess of alcohol in the system. Other tastes that clients experience are that of special foods which, like all the other senses, may trigger past emotional memories.

SENSING REIKI SPIRITUALLY

The system of Reiki is a spiritual practice even though a large part of its focus in contemporary society is on hands-on healing. This focus does not negate the spiritual aspects of the system; spirituality is innate in any true healing practice. The National Center for Complementary and Alternative Medicine (NCCAM) includes spiritual practices such as Reiki in their research by defining spirituality as "an individual's sense of purpose and meaning to life, beyond material values. Spirituality may be practiced in many ways, including through religion."

Spiritually, you can sense Reiki. This is not unlike sensing with any of the other major sense organs. The five sense organs are physical while to be spiritually oriented is to be open to sensing the wonders of the world, many of them intangible. As you float deep inside the universe during your treatment, or experience a high that is clear and light, you are touching something inside that you have been ignoring or do not often notice. Reiki offers you a keyhole glimpse into these spaces that you can enter. It aids you in becoming more open to your inner healing.

A Healthy Spirit

If our spirit is healthy and conformed to the truth, the body will get healthy naturally.

Reiki Ryôhô Hikkei
Usui Reiki Ryôhô Gakkai

Your spiritual side is the one that searches for a deeper understanding of your role in the world. When you respond spiritually during a Reiki treatment you trigger a search for spiritual fulfillment in your self. This might include:
- Realizing there is a state of inner happiness in contrast to happiness gained solely from material wealth.

- Sensing a natural connection to life and a personal responsibility to its ongoing balance.
- Acknowledging the wisdom of your inner truth.
- Recognizing that enlightenment is possible and that it resides within.

You may find yourself searching out more peaceful ways of being, changing habits that have worked against you living a healthy and happy life. Your perceptions about life may alter. You may become inspired to begin studying other spiritual and/or religious practices and take up yoga, or qi gong.

The Universe and You

Jasmine had been enjoying her Reiki treatments enormously. Her plan was to continue with one treatment a week until she felt she had moved through the unmotivated slump she had recently been in. The Reiki treatments were helping and by the fourth treatment she was totally into it. She lay on the treatment table, prepared to go deep down into herself as she normally did, when all of a sudden it felt as if her physical body had disappeared. Jasmine seemed to expand, that was the only word she could think of to describe this weird sensation. It was a little frightening and she grabbed at the edge of the table to steady herself, bringing back her sense of physicality. After a while she let go and relaxed and it seemed as if she was in some big black space which curiously also had an aspect of lightness about it. That treatment was a turning point in Jasmine's life, she went on to discover a major part of her life that she had been ignoring; her spirituality.

As you heal, your spirituality comes to the fore for you to explore it further.

No Sensations During Your Treatment

Expectations may have built up prior to arriving at your Reiki session. Some reports regarding treatments are amazing and even hard to believe if you haven't experienced it for yourself.

Reiki treatments are not always "out there". It is possible to lie down on the treatment table and have a lovely relaxing treatment without any overt unearthly experiences. This can be disappointing if you had expected flashing lights and spooky sensations. Others tend to relate the amazing things that they experience, not the less interesting aspects such as "it was pleasant".

Reiki is not like taking a pill. Nothing is guaranteed; not healing, not sensation – nothing. And neither is it necessary to feel anything during a Reiki treatment.

Your response depends upon many factors, not all of them rational or tangible.

Your state of mind is an important factor. If you do not feel open to the treatment or you are uncomfortable, it is unlikely that you draw on a great deal of energy. Many clients realize this when at their second treatment they give over to a greater extent and the benefits flow freer.

Your energetic awareness may also be limited. Society has never taught you to be aware of yourself energetically. You may have been labeled silly as a child if you sensed something intangible. To reunite with this knowledge can take some practice and it can be thrilling to build this innate quality consciously.

Your relationship with the Reiki practitioner is integral to your experience. Being wary of your practitioner or uncomfortable in her presence means that your focus during the treatment is not directed at self-healing. In this case, you cannot support your growing consciousness.

The practitioner's own energetic limits are also a factor in your experience. If she has not spent time developing her energetic strength, her ability to move energy through her body is restricted. Obstacles within obstruct the free flow of energy and must be gradually worked away at by the practitioner in order that she become the best conduit for it. Only then can you draw on significant amounts of energy. The practitioner's intent is a part of this process and it must be clear and grounded at each treatment for the treatment to be most effective.

If the environment is right and the practitioner professional and experienced, then you must accept whatever the treatment brings or doesn't bring and know that this is Reiki. By aligning with the basic philosophy of Reiki all you need do in your treatment is to learn to let go of expected outcomes. This attitude will domino throughout your life and you will find yourself moving more smoothly through any bumps that you may encounter.

THE END OF YOUR TREATMENT

The Reiki treatment is over. You begin to focus more on your immediate surroundings and are gently helped up and off the treatment table by your Reiki practitioner.

Your practitioner hands you a glass of water to help support the clearing process that your body is experiencing. Curiously many clients find that their mouths become dry during and/or after a treatment. This is a part of, or the journey back to, your original balance.

Water is a natural cleanser, within and without the human form. In the microcosm of human form, fluid moves through you to transport goodness from one place to another and to wash out that which you no longer require; sending it elsewhere where nature has always had further use for it. In your renewed state of balance a stronger connection with life's natural co-existence is emphasized. Your human form has multiple roles within this wheel of life and being a receptacle, and filter, for fluid is just one of them. In the macrocosm, water completes the same cycle as it falls from the skies and cleanses the world, washing it clean, transporting goodness and waste through nature's homelands.

The practitioner is your guide to processing your Reiki treatment. He may ask about your experience during the treatment to determine if there is a way that he can support you. He, in turn, may discuss your treatment in terms of what he felt but does not interpret this.

He may mention the possibility of future treatments (if he deems them to be helpful), as well as the possibility that you may experience a cleansing process and answer any questions regarding your treatment or future treatments.

Your practitioner may also offer you supportive practices that you can involve yourself with at home. This could include a simple meditation practice to help promote the clearing of your energy to create balance. Continuing with a meditation or technique is an excellent idea for at least two reasons. One is that it helps you to regain your balance quicker. The second is that conscious self-healing is the next step up the ladder as far as improving your health and quality of life. Taking self-responsibility for your health is the missing link for many healing practices. If the client can become involved and work together with the practitioner then the speed and quality of the healing can be vastly improved in a natural way.

DIAGNOSING WITH REIKI

A Reiki practitioner does not diagnose. A Reiki practitioner does not need to diagnose; energy is the true healer. The concept of distinguishing or identifying a disease, or the cause of a disease, with Reiki is inappropriate. Reiki is energy and the practitioner is a receptacle for that energy. This equation does not hold in it the need for, or the acquired ability to, diagnose.

The benefits of this are numerous. The energy, Reiki, is allowed to do what it needs at an unconscious level without a practitioner or client identifying an issue, cause or disease and attempting to deal with it. This takes away the concept of human error so that a practitioner who does not know you intimately cannot make presumptions about your life from an uninformed perspective. Always question whether anyone has the right to direct you in your life choices. If a practitioner is incorrect in her diagnosis or interpretation this can ultimately be unempowering.

It is often in times of turmoil that a client turns to a treatment such as Reiki to try to sort her life out. Practitioners must be aware that such a client is extremely vulnerable and any suggestions that are offered may be taken very seriously and acted upon.

The Ultimate Truth Lies Within

Jane knew nothing about the system of Reiki. She visited a Healing Festival with a friend and took advantage of a free 10-minute Reiki treatment where she was told by the practitioner that she had an entity attached to her leg. Jane felt scared and that night began to feel strange sensations in her leg. Jane visited another Reiki practitioner to seek further advice regarding this frightening entity. The professional Reiki practitioner explained that the entity had never existed but that the previous practitioner may have felt something energetic at the leg and interpreted the sensation in that way. Jane received a wonderful Reiki treatment and was no longer bothered by "her" entity.

A Reiki practitioner may begin to diagnose if she is lacking in confidence or insecure with her Reiki practice. If, through inexperience, she cannot comprehend that the energy works best without her intervention then she is likely to try to make something happen by directing the energy and then telling the client what she has done and what that entails. This is not Reiki, no matter how well intentioned the motives of the practitioner are. Sometimes the "power" of one's Reiki ability can create a false confidence.

There are manipulative forms of energy work that claim to be able to direct and diagnose energy but the system of Reiki is not one of them.

The Snake-oil Merchant

Christine and James had been trying to start a family. Christine decided to learn Reiki and had just finished her course when she became pregnant. Unfortunately for Christine it was not yet to be a reality and she had a miscarriage. Not long after, she met a Reiki teacher who claimed to know what her problem was and how to fix it. The practitioner told Christine that she had been wrongly "attuned" to her left ovary during her Reiki course and assured Christine that she could fix it – for a tidy sum; claiming that Christine would then be able to successfully fall pregnant.

This kind of action is not about empowering the client; it is about holding power over the client. Christine sensed the practitioner's behavior was unethical and did not follow through with his advice. She confirmed with her Reiki teacher that Reiki does not "attune" you to anything, especially body parts, and a Reiki practitioner cannot ensure that you become pregnant.

A Reiki practitioner should direct you to look within for the answers you require, rather than encouraging you to search for them from others. You have all the knowledge inside you and when you connect with it, your healing is all the more profound.

Referring You on to Another Therapy

Although Reiki treatments are advertised as being suitable for anyone of any age, in any shape, of any sex, culture or religion, there are times when your Reiki practitioner should refer you on to another health care worker. This is not to say that a Reiki treatment would not be beneficial but there may be a more immediate need that it is appropriate to take care of first.

Reiki practitioners are obviously not trained counselors, physicians, acupuncturists, homeopaths, dieticians etc… (unless specified otherwise), however, your Reiki practitioner may have a list of health care workers that he can refer you on to. His reasons for doing so may be that you require medical treatment or that you do not appear to be responding to Reiki in a manner that is satisfactory to you and/or him.

An example of this is if a client has a serious mental health issue but has not yet received medical attention. In this situation a Reiki practitioner should first refer the client on to a mental health worker. Another example might occur after a Reiki treatment when a serious issue has come to the surface and the client feels the need to be able to talk this issue out with a professional. In this case, the Reiki practitioner should refer the client on to a professional counselor or psychotherapist.

A client may always receive Reiki in conjunction with any other therapy or medical treatment according to the principal understandings of Reiki. It is always good practice for a Reiki practitioner to ask the client to inform his other health worker/s that he is also receiving Reiki treatments.

A Reiki practitioner should never discourage you from seeking medical advice. A medical doctor provides primary health care and, unlike a Reiki practitioner, is educated to be able to discuss with, and advise, the client as to the possible treatment options. Ultimately, it is always the client's choice; yet, the Reiki practitioner must work within the boundaries set by society.

Finding the Right Help

Michael was recently separated from his wife and not coping. When he arrived at his Reiki treatment, all he felt like doing was talking. He didn't realize it until he sat down and it all started flooding out; in the end he only received a brief 10-minute Reiki treatment. Michael booked in for a Reiki treatment the following week and the same scenario occurred. The Reiki practitioner who was not a qualified counselor suggested to Michael that he book in for a session with a local counselor first. Michael took the Reiki practitioner's advice. Working with the counselor he found that he could more effectively process the thoughts that were bothering him. Michael soon returned for some more Reiki treatments and was now able to appreciate the peace and tranquility they offered him.

Part III

Post-Treatment

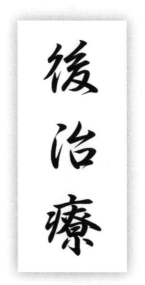

YOUR PRACTITIONER'S
POST-TREATMENT RESPONSIBILITY

Now that your session is finished, is the actual Reiki treatment finished?

As previously discussed your Reiki practitioner has a duty of care to you as the client. The standard of care that a practitioner should provide is comparable to that required of professionals generally, and to medical practitioners in particular.[27] This includes fully informing you of any aspects that may relate to your treatment but fall outside of the time that you and the practitioner spend together during the session.

Your practitioner will have notified you at the beginning of your session about the cleansing process that works hand-in-hand with the system of Reiki; this is your body's own natural healing process which Reiki stimulates and supports.

Your Reiki treatment has initiated a process and for that reason your Reiki practitioner should make certain that she gives you the resources to deal with it. This will include suggesting how to approach and comprehend the cleansing process. She will also offer you the opportunity to contact her if you need to discuss anything relating to your post treatment experience. If you wish to contact your Reiki practitioner by telephone, this should occur during working hours. Email is an alternative communication method for practitioners and clients that, if used professionally, can be quick and effective. If you need to actually see the practitioner it is expected that you pay for your practitioner's time, in the same way that you would any therapist.

Your practitioner will also have discussed how she can support you further on your healing journey. From your shared discussions after the treatment your practitioner may have suggested further treatments to support the changes you wish to make, or referred you on to another therapist or health care worker. She may also have discussed the possibility of you developing your self-healing ability with a Reiki course.

It is possible that your practitioner may teach you some simple practices to follow-up your treatment with at home, on the proviso that you return in a week or two. She may simply suggest that you come back for another treatment the next time you feel the need for some serious relaxation. Together, you will have planned the most beneficial course for you to take and it is up to both of you to follow through with your agreements.

Are You a Satisfied Customer?

If you are dissatisfied with your Reiki treatment you can, and should, make a complaint. Initially, it is best to contact the practitioner herself and try to resolve the problem. If you feel that you need to take your issue further you may contact the practitioner's clinic or department head, association, insurance company, national body or relevant authority. All complaints should be set out in writing. Do be aware that your Reiki practitioner will also be notified of your complaint. A Complaints Procedure will be available from any professional organization for you to follow and to ensure that your voice is heard.

If you wish to offer positive feedback about your experience this can also be provided to your practitioner, the practitioner's clinic, association and/or national body.

DISORIENTATION AFTER A TREATMENT

What a treatment! You leave the clinic, hop into your car and can't remember where the steering wheel is. This scenario is unrealistic but it is undeniable that a Reiki treatment can be quite disorienting. It is possible that you may feel light-headed, sleepy and unable to make quick judgments after a treatment. In the last hour you went from everyday mental activity to a relaxed state where you opened yourself up to allow your body's natural healing abilities to take over and run the show. After coming out of that state, you are now trying to function as you did before. Is this possible?

Your body needs to re-balance itself. Interestingly, you will find that this re-balancing continues over the next few days and even weeks – if you consciously support its process. Most importantly, you will need to readjust to everyday life to be able to get from your treatment to your next appointment, work or home.

To bring yourself out of deep relaxation, your practitioner will offer you a glass of water to support your cleansing process. As the water washes down through you, you begin to feel refreshed. You shake yourself out of your slumber. Maybe your world looks and feels slightly different. Your practitioner gently discusses your treatment and in this communicative process your senses are activated back to their regular functioning level.

There are a number of activities you need to be careful about doing after your treatment. One is driving. If you plan to drive immediately after your treatment think twice before hopping in behind that steering wheel. To be a safe driver you need to be 100% aware of your surroundings. You would not want to have had a wonderful Reiki treatment only to end up in a traffic accident.

The other action to be careful of is going back to work. If you need to use any complicated machinery or you have planned an important meeting just after your Reiki treatment it may be wiser to either change your treatment appointment to after work or reschedule work that may not require your immediate full attention. Work is often hectic, with no time to relax and treasure that thread of inner connectedness that you have begun nurturing. Sometimes, the best thing to do is to go home and relax in the garden or just to go to bed.

Unfortunately you cannot always relax for as long as you would like at a professional clinic after your treatment. Your practitioner most likely has another client arriving soon and the room needs to be prepared. If your practitioner does not think that you are ready to drive or work machinery, he may offer some suggestions. These could include resting in the waiting room, if there is one. Spend some time there after the treatment before moving out onto the street. Otherwise, you could go to a local café and enjoy a fruit juice or tea as you readjust. While there, you can enjoy contemplating your session and maybe life in general.

Grounding after a Treatment

If you still find that you are light-headed after having a drink and a rest you can perform this small exercise. Visualize a large ball of energy in your head moving down through you to your hara center (just below your navel), down along your legs and into the Earth. This exercise will ground your energy into the energy of the Earth enabling you to feel calm, clear and aware.

Your Body and the Cleansing Process

Throughout *Your Reiki Treatment* there has been reference to the body's ability to heal itself. Your body has its own natural way of dealing with illness and impurities. Scientifically, it has been shown that energy becomes more active in areas that are not functioning as effectively as they should. This is the body busying itself at self-healing and may be sensed by both the client and practitioner. This busy-ness may also trigger the cleansing process; a further development that the energy takes to support healing of the body.

A Reiki treatment offers energy to the client's body for it to draw on, to clear the client's energy. This helps the client's body strengthen its own reserves and work toward a renewed balance. Inline with this concept it is often felt that an illness may get "worse" before it gets better. An example of this can be seen in the functioning of one of the body's warning systems – fever. Most fevers are thought to support the natural healing process (except for those considered "maladaptive"); with fever being triggered once the body senses inflammation.[28] Fever shakes your immune system awake to start healing. Once the original inflammation reduces and is out of the red zone, the fever subsides – its warning signals are no longer needed. Here the term "worse" is relative to the situation and the ultimate result.

In the same way, when the energy is busy stimulating your inner healing, a cleansing process may be set in motion. This is the body removing that which it no longer needs. The magic of Reiki is that it actually supports it, in contrast to the confusion created by adding medications to your system. Medications only give the body more to sort out and deal with on top of the initial problem.

Cleansing is a natural and positive experience. The human body has gradually adjusted itself through natural selection to be the ultimate self-healing tool. Imagine that at every moment in your life your body is trying to bring itself back into balance, shifting energy and stimulating you in physical, and non-physical, ways to allow you to operate as a healthier and more effective individual. Reiki simply supports this process in working more effectively.

A clearing may take place during the treatment itself or after the session. It may come in all shapes and sizes. You might experience heightened emotions, physical reactions like getting a cold or even have unusual dreams.

Jason's Dreamtime

Jason is a Reiki practitioner who is highly aware of when his self-healing practices initiate major change. At these times his body begins to clear itself. He doesn't feel this physically; instead he has unusual dreams. In a dream he might be walking in the street when, suddenly, he finds himself pulling lumps of wood out of his hands. Or he is dreaming that he is talking to a friend and hot metal pours out of his ears. Jason's dream clearings express themselves as the physical removal of human fluids or natural elements. He doesn't mind because he understands that the dreams are affirming that his self-healing practices are working.

It is important that you don't set yourself up to believe that these clearing effects will occur, as that may result in them occurring needlessly. You will receive whatever you need and you should not become attached to that or fear it.

When you receive a Reiki treatment, you are consciously stimulating the clearing and, therefore, you are at some level in charge of what is happening. If you find that the clearing is too unpleasant for you then you can decide to stop the healing process by halting treatments, and closing your mind to healing and change. Your body will return to its old habits and your innate processes will continue their uphill struggle without your conscious support.

Your Body's Natural Clearing Process

No-one should put themselves in a position where they feel they can no longer handle it and everyone must remember that there is no ulterior force at work here – there is just you and you are in control. Take your power.

The Japanese Art of Reiki
Bronwen and Frans Stiene

THE PHYSICAL CLEANSING PROCESS

Working with Reiki stimulates your natural healing ability with the resulting clearings often becoming more apparent. This could be due to you exhibiting a higher level of consciousness toward the entire process. It may also be due to your energetic flow building in strength. You are more open and, therefore, greater clearing is allowed to occur. It is as if you are clearing out a clogged-up water pipe. When the pipe becomes clearer, the easier it is for the rushing water to flow through and further clean it out. This is cyclical in nature and gradually the energy becomes more substantial and the healing more effective.

As your body's energy regains its freer flow, it is quite common to experience an obvious physical reaction. For example, if you have tense shoulders your body has miraculously thought of ways to accommodate this imbalance. It tightens up elsewhere and pulls somewhere else. Your body is now functioning in a totally new, although unnatural, position; it is managing with a false sense of balance due to your tight shoulder muscles. When your shoulder muscles loosen during a Reiki treatment your body attempts to re-balance itself. This may create aches and pains during the treatment as well as after the treatment as the body processes the energetic experience. The repercussions of a Reiki treatment can be like touching the thread of a spiderweb, with its consequent reverberations throughout the whole web. You can stand back and watch the web and it will continue to vibrate until the entire web has resettled itself. So it is with the body's cleansing process; touch it and its effect will resound throughout each fiber of your body, finally settling you back into in a new, healthier position.

Removing Pain

Bob, a football player, booked in for a Reiki treatment to help ease the pain in his leg. For two days after the treatment he noticed that his leg had a slight spasm and was shaking, which it had never done before. He decided to take it easy and wait to see what would eventuate. Once the spasms and shaking disappeared, so did his pain.

A dormant physical issue can be brought to light by receiving a Reiki treatment. A painful kidney stone, for example, may be noticed after a treatment. Your body may be attempting to remove the stone as a part of your cleansing process. This is not dangerous but you do need to be aware and grounded when making judgments regarding your health status. In such a situation it is highly recommended that you organize a visit to your primary health care worker to observe the kidney stone's progress. A Reiki practitioner does not have the knowledge, skills or tools to be able to do this. You may, however, continue with the Reiki treatments while your kidney stone remains under observation to support its natural passing through your system.

Another client experienced pain in her chest during a Reiki treatment. Wisely, she immediately booked herself in for an ECG only to find out there was nothing wrong. A physical response of clearing may also be the result of an emotional release; a physical problem does not need to be at the root of a physical clearing. A visit to your primary health care worker is always recommended if there are health concerns and this should be wholeheartedly supported by your practitioner.

Am I Okay?

Patricia enjoyed her Reiki treatment enormously. Afterward, she realized that she had begun to menstruate heavily. It was the wrong time of the month and she was concerned. She approached her practitioner and asked if everything was okay. Her practitioner explained that it should be seen as a healthy experience as it was a physical clearing of the body initiated by the Reiki. However, if it continued or concerned Patricia excessively she should definitely visit her primary health care worker for a check up.

This clearing process is constant, though not always perceptible and not always recognized for what it is – a re-balancing of the body. Some of the physical clearing responses you may experience are vomiting, pains in the limbs, flu-like symptoms, diarrhea or headaches.

The Non-Physical Cleansing Process

There are numerous understandings of what a non-physical clearing may be. It could be the release of emotions, a clearer sense of purpose, and deep beneath it all is the potential to make inroads in your own spiritual development.

According to the Usui Reiki Ryôhô Gakkai manual[29], on being asked what the system of Reiki was, Usui Mikao is quoted as replying that "First we have to heal our spirit."

Spiritual practices have at their foundation the concept of clearing because clearing the body is a natural and connected method that supports healthy living. A spiritual practice utilizes the concept of connection as a universal law and the practice's underpinnings must work in alignment with this. Your spirituality resides in you, and in everything you think and do. It is difficult to place a finger on but humans know when something is not right as well as when it is absolutely perfect.

Humanity has always had a deep longing to connect completely with its ancestry; be that human, animal, plant or something intangible and unseen. Humans originated from the planet earth millions of years ago, and the earth originated from the universe and before that ... we do not know. It is the desire to link back to our origins, to find that source within ourselves that drives us to practice methods like meditation, yoga, qi gong and Reiki. We are looking for a deeper way to heal so that we can be at One with that which came before. This is not a new thought. Spiritual connectivity is a part of life and forms the rhythm of the planet, long before we decided that the planet should live in rhythm with us.

Removing the clutter from your spiritual being is a part of the cleansing process and this clutter is not always physical. A non-physical clearing may often be found at the base of a physical clearing.

The Heart Response

Jana experienced a clearing that she described like this: "During the treatment I had certain feelings depending upon where your hands were on my body. At my heart I felt so sad as I remembered a bad situation I was involved in with my old boyfriend. Also, when you were at the same place on my back, I almost felt like crying." The day after the treatment Jana called to tell the practitioner that when she got home she had a good cry and had gained some incredible insights into her past relationship. She was feeling a little shook up but definitely much clearer and happier. Jana had gotten herself back on her own spiritual path; she could feel that she was now in a better place.

Being able to clear yourself of clogged up emotions and thoughts is an amazing natural ability. Don't allow your energy to be stuck, it could be stopping your emotional connection to life. To stop the tears is to stop the energy. Be in touch with your emotions and recognize their validity as essential to your humanness.

During a Reiki treatment a sense of your original connection to life might be rekindled, reminding you of the universal law that you cannot change anything that has happened in the past; it is done. Society today expects us to hold on to our lives, those around us and our belongings with great emotional attachment. This mental attitude is an extra challenge to living healthy and balanced lives. To sense your connection anew can help relieve some of the stresses that society places upon you.

Some of the non-physical clearings that you may experience are crying, feeling buoyed one day and depressed the next, anger, dreams, sadness, a reminder of your disconnected state, and fear. Past trauma might also re-surface or you may re-experience grief over the death of a loved one.

Reiki practitioners recommend that you continue with your treatment to move through your clearings and if you and your practitioner feel that it is appropriate you can also be referred on to another health care worker.

LENGTH OF THE CLEANSING PROCESS

Some Reiki teachings work with the understanding that there are 21 days of clearing after a Reiki treatment. Each Reiki treatment that you receive certainly has the potential to initiate a palpable cleansing process within you and the concept of 21 days is a traditional timeline to create change within.

Cleansing is an innate process and one that is always at work but your conscious acknowledgement of it may only have been awakened at the touch of your Reiki treatment.

Accepting the concept of self-healing is, in itself, a personal journey; it is quite different to the concept of conventional western medicine. Self-healing is not greatly encouraged in those circles – yet. There the focus is on cure and sometimes prevention. The system of Reiki works with the convention that true prevention is looking for ways to support your body in its self-healing process and Reiki can aid you in that.

Accepting Alternative Practices in the Mainstream

The mainstream has treated them [healing approaches that incorporate emotional and spiritual elements] like poor stepchildren and relegated them to the fringes of alternative medicine. The argument that they are untested, and therefore can't be taken seriously, is not valid. I'm afraid that we are holding the alternative therapies, those that use mind-body and spiritual techniques, to a higher standard than we apply to mainstream medicine.

Molecules of Emotion
Candace B. Pert, Ph.D.

Receiving Reiki treatments does not mean that you will never get sick. In fact, it encourages the body to remove its impurities; viewing the body as being in a constant state of imbalance. A cleansing process might be short or long depending on what is happening within you. No matter where you are on your spiritual journey you will experience shifts. It is not a failure to undergo a cleansing process, if anything it can be courageous to totally give over to that inherent ability and to face it consciously instead of letting it work away at a snail's pace in the background.

In the beginning these shifts might seem uncomfortable and confronting but the deeper you move into your self-healing, the more faith you have in your own aptitude to deal with these issues as you become more balanced. An answer to moving through tough patches can be to receive more Reiki treatments.

The more Reiki you are exposed to, the deeper the cleansing process. If it becomes too uncomfortable then you will need to adapt the number of treatments or the regularity of the treatments you are undertaking. It is possible to overdo energy work. Some clients become so enthusiastic about the changes they experience that they push too hard. Working with Reiki is comparable to working out in the gym. Attending the gym three times a day and attempting to lift more than you can handle leaves you feeling wrecked the following day. Always be compassionate to yourself, show respect to your body by listening to it. Avail yourself of other health care workers whenever you and your practitioner believe that it might be beneficial to your self development.

NO APPARENT CLEANSING PROCESS

It is not necessary to have any kind of "symptoms" during, or after, a Reiki treatment. Not ostensibly undergoing a cleansing process does not infer that the treatment did not work.

Most importantly, no two people have the same energetic levels. Your energy is as specific to you as your fingerprint. Energy is so subtle and subjective that to claim that one level could be exactly the same as another is highly illogical. Your life experience is unique and has affected every facet of your life, including your energetic being, in an incomparable way. For example, after a Reiki course a student may have begun to sense a tingling in his hands – thinking it is normal, while another may not, although both may have sat the same Reiki training. Therefore, what an individual may sense and expect will be specific to that person's cultural and personal background.

There will be many reasons why one may not initially sense anything at, or after, a Reiki treatment. The truth is that most of humanity is still relatively disconnected from its true nature. This may change with time when working with Reiki. As the client gradually transforms, the more open he becomes to the concept of self-healing with Reiki and the easier it is to place his consciousness with his healing potential.

A Knock at the Door

Jessica had been diagnosed with Chronic Fatigue Syndrome by her doctor. At her first Reiki treatment she could sense absolutely nothing and began to wonder if Reiki did anything at all. The practitioner, too, felt that Jessica's body was unresponsive. He knew that he had to let go of his attachment to want to sense something during a treatment and from his extensive Reiki experience he knew that the Reiki was possibly working at a very subtle level preparing Jessica to open up to it, if she continued with the treatments.

After a number of treatments Jessica did begin to open up and let the energy be drawn by her body. She said she felt as if previously the energy had been knocking at the door but she couldn't let it in until the appropriate moment. Her practitioner was thankful that Jessica had been patient with the process. After quite a few months of receiving treatments Jessica's attitude and physical strength started to improve. She found that she was responding in many individual ways to the treatments both during and after them. Jessica also discovered that there is a whole art to receiving.

Even if you believe you are not responding to your treatments, after a number of treatments stop and look back objectively at your life. Have there been any changes? You will undoubtedly be able to see developments with certain things having fallen away. Just because you didn't experience sudden and dramatic change does not mean that it has not occurred. Perhaps your fear has lessened or the pain in your arm is gone. A useful way to compare your life's change and to reflect upon the effects of Reiki is through journaling. Keep a journal of your daily thoughts, feelings and dreams. If you are seriously working toward change this is where you will find fascinating reading in a month or two.

How regularly you receive a treatment will make a difference. The closer together, the greater the potential for change to occur. Your connection with your practitioner is also an important factor in your treatment and your attitude to the treatment. Your intent during a treatment and your commitment to self-healing will affect your experience.

To Drink or Not to Drink

Genevieve was a drinker. She loved to drink. As she got older she realized that she could no longer deal with the great amounts of alcohol she was imbibing. She was advised that a Reiki treatment might help her lessen her intake. The night before the treatment she got pretty smashed as usual and even though she enjoyed the Reiki treatment it did not feel particularly effective. That afternoon she went home and poured herself a nice big drink.

Relying on a practitioner to change your life will never work, the only person you can ever rely on to heal you is yourself. The more that you work on yourself with an energetic practice the easier it will become for you to sense.

The Number of Treatments Required

A Reiki practitioner cannot tell you how many Reiki treatments you will require at any point of your experience. This is your decision to make in conjunction with professional advice from the practitioner.

Most importantly you need to assess what your requirements were and are. Did you attend the Reiki session for the purposes of a one-off relaxation therapy or was your intention to delve deeper into self-healing? Once you are clear as to your intention you can then decide what your next strategic step toward a healthier and more balanced life will be.

Within the Reiki community it is often suggested that three treatments, close together, will help a client to move through any acute issues. These treatments might be once a day or once a week but not spaced much further apart than that. However, there are no rules with this energetic practice and three treatments may be too little or too many for you at this moment in your life. If there are major issues that you would like to work on with Reiki then it would naturally be recommended that you continue with the treatments until you feel that you have moved through those issues.

In the Jungle, Beware the Lion

Shanti, an avid meditator, had rheumatoid arthritis. At her first Reiki treatment she explained that she knew she was heading into a difficult period as her joints were starting to stiffen and swell.

"Last night I had a bad dream. When I get very sick I dream terrible dreams and am chased by wild animals. Once a crow flew to my head and threw dirty water all over me. Last night, I dreamt a lion was chasing me. I was screaming so loudly my husband had to shake me awake."

During most of the treatment, she lay with her eyes open, obviously nervous. Toward its end she began to loosen up a little. Afterward, she said she had felt energy moving in her legs, hands and stomach. The practitioner and Shanti decided upon three consecutive sessions of Reiki to see if they could stimulate Shanti's own self-healing abilities.

Shanti entered the second treatment much more relaxed and snored lightly throughout. At the end of the treatment she related her previous night's dream. "The wild lion was chasing me again and this time I scrabbled around and found mud to throw at him, before running away."

At the third treatment, Shanti remarked that she was feeling much better already. "Last night something different happened, too. In my dream I was in the jungle and I could hear the lion. I didn't run away. For the first time I calmly looked around and picked up some great big rocks and threw them at him like this." Shanti demonstrated throwing a heavy boulder with all her might. "And the lion ran away!"

Feeling satisfied with her rapid progress, she was happy to continue with her meditation work at home now. If she ever found herself in a similar state again, she said she would come back for some more Reiki.

Sometimes setting an aim of three sessions can be an excellent goal for you and your practitioner to work toward. Whatever you decide together, make sure that you feel comfortable with it.

Phyllis Lei Furumoto, granddaughter of the woman who brought the system of Reiki to the West, said that her grandmother, Hawayo Takata, would not treat people who could not commit to receiving a treatment every day for 30 consecutive days. That level of commitment and strength of intent on the behalf of both the client and practitioner assures that whatever can be done, will be done.

If the practitioner feels that it is suitable for you, she may recommend that you also learn the system of Reiki so that you can begin to physically and mentally take more responsibility for the state of your health. If you become a Reiki practitioner, you are still welcome to enjoy Reiki treatments.

Bulk Reiki Treatments

Do not pay for "bulk" treatments before you are sure that the practitioner, and the Reiki treatments themselves, are what you are looking for. Experience these aspects before making any decisions about future treatments.

ASSISTING YOUR SELF-HEALING AT HOME

After receiving a Reiki treatment, it is beneficial if you can continue moving the energy yourself at home. Even though you may not have completed a Reiki course, everyone can heal themselves and what you need most of all is the clear intent to do so.

Healing is Innate

Providing a Reiki treatment can also serve as a demonstration for the client, an opportunity to try to introduce something they can do for themselves at home, adding a sense of empowerment and extending the treatment scope. For even without training, using the hand positions can be a quieting and calming event that may allow the client to refocus at a time of stress. If the process of using Reiki at home resonates with the client, they too can take the initial training course to enhance their ability, thereby increasing their sense of commitment to their growth, change, and sense of self.

The Use of Reiki in Psychotherapy
Mary Ann LaTorre

If you wish to create a follow-up routine to your Reiki treatment to keep the energy moving and to ensure that you continue to take responsibility for yourself here are some tips. Choose one or two of these practices to create your own daily healing routine.

1. Meditate

Ask your practitioner for a meditation which you can perform for up to 15 minutes a day. There are a number of meditations taught within the system of Reiki and your practitioner will be able to advise which is the best for you. Research into one simple form of meditation has had over 500 studies completed on its physiological, psychological, and sociological effects. It has been found that through meditation there are improved mental abilities, improved health including reduced stress and anxiety, reduced hospitalization, reduced incidence of disease, increased longevity and improved social behavior such as improved self-confidence, family life, relationships and job satisfaction, while reducing anxiety.[30]

Choose a good time of the day for practicing, perhaps first thing in the morning or before going to bed.

2. Journaling

Journaling means to write in a journal. It can be difficult to find someone to share your thoughts with on the many intimate subjects or issues that may arise from your Reiki experience. Writing them down can be a huge relief and release. It can be a very beneficial way to express yourself without the judgments of others. By writing in a journal there are no boundaries. Ideally, it is best to write every day in a journal even if it is only a line or two. The habit is a wonderful one to begin and pursue.

3. Hands-on Healing

Naturally, an important part of the system of Reiki is hands-on healing. This is easy to do at home though it can take a little confidence building to work well with it.

Gentle touch in itself is highly effective with one research paper evaluating the effectiveness and safety of healing by gentle touch. It stated that the healing that ensued was associated with improved psychological and physical functioning in the majority of subjects.[31]

To perform hands-on healing place your hands next to each other, or even on top of each other if you wish, at the place where you feel emotionally stuck or have physical pain. Set your intent that you are going to do healing on yourself and don't forget your intent – that you are open to receive whatever it is that you may need at this exact moment in your life.

GROUNDING YOURSELF

To further your self-practice you can also learn some basic grounding techniques that work with the hara region which is three finger widths below your navel, inside your body. These techniques will help you deal with everyday life in a balanced way and will support your Reiki treatments. They will help you to feel grounded and safe and secure within yourself. Working with the hara is a good first self-development step as it is the foundation of most Japanese energetic practices.

As the system of Reiki is a Japanese practice that was created in the early 1900s it originally worked with the hara. This area of the body was considered to be the center of the body's energetic powerhouse. Many martial arts and Ki practices that were formalized in Japan at the same time as the system of Reiki such as karate, judo and aikidô also work with the hara region.

The word hara literally means stomach, abdomen or belly in Japanese. Energy is stored at this point from where it expands throughout the whole body. This is the energy you are born with, the energy that is the essence of your life and gives you your life's purpose and stamina. It is not just the energy that you receive from your parents when you are conceived but most importantly it is the energetic connection between you and universal energy.

In traditional Japanese teachings and exercises today the hara system is still the main focus for building a person's energy. Reestablishing your connection through the hara will ensure good health and recovery from illness. Working at this point of the body ensures access to a reliable source of strength whenever needed.

Think of the hara as your grounding point. From this central point there is an ability to cope with everyday tasks and sudden emergencies with an ease of understanding. This allows appropriate action to be taken in a balanced and unprejudiced manner.

Include one of these grounding techniques into your daily routine.

Strengthening your Hara Connection I

- Sit comfortably with your back naturally straight.
- Close your eyes.
- Breathe in through your nose and out through your mouth. As you breathe in feel the energy entering your nostrils and move it down to your hara center.
- Keep your awareness there and hold it for a moment.
- Slowly breathe out through your mouth.
- Repeat this breathing cycle for as long as you wish.
- If you find it difficult to bring your breath all the way down to your hara you can place one or both of your hands on the hara center to aid the mental focus, then try again.

Strengthening your Hara Connection II

- Stand relaxed with your feet slightly apart and your eyes partially closed.
- Place your hands above your head, middle fingers touching with your palms facing the floor.
- Slowly push the energy down the front of the body toward your hara center.
- Place your hands gently over the hara and let them rest for a while.
- Feel the energy build in your hands and body.

REIKI AND MASSAGE

The system of Reiki is simple; it is based on fundamental universal laws and does not try to manipulate or diagnose. For these reasons many practitioners combine it with other therapies.

Spas have become a popular aspect of the fashion culture and within that there are many therapies available. No longer do you just get a facial and a Swedish massage but thermal mud baths, honey treatments, herbal remedies, hot stone therapy and much more have been created to tempt, relax and revive. You will find that Reiki has been added to many of these spa therapies and treatments as an extra luxury. You may not even be aware that you are receiving Reiki as it may be added, almost imperceptibly, to the therapy smorgasbord.

Reiki and massage are occasionally spoken of in the same breath as if they are one and the same or sometimes you might even hear of a Reiki Massage. There's even a practice today called Reiki-ssage™.

The truth is that Reiki and massage can be combined very well and yet are two very separate practices.

Similarities between the two largely exist in how you experience the set-up of the sessions. A Reiki session in its entirety is approximately the same length of time as a massage – it may take one hour or a little more or less. An individual practitioner or therapist treats you, yet it is also possible to have multiple practitioners or therapists working on you. The cost of the session is also comparable as you are paying for the trained practitioner or therapist's time, experience and qualifications.

Another similarity between the two treatments is that they are both touch based even though the actual manner of using touch is drastically different.

The differences between the two practices are also quite notable. Reiki is not manipulative; it does not intentionally move any parts of your body. You do not remove any clothing for a Reiki treatment. No oils or other tools are utilized during a Reiki treatment except for the practitioner's hands which are laid gently on or just off the client's body. Reiki is therefore also non-intrusive.

You may find that many massage therapists have studied Reiki and will include it at the beginning or end of a massage or if there is a particular body part that they feel may benefit from Reiki. For example a very stiff muscle that is too sore to manipulate might well receive Reiki from a massage therapist. A therapist's hands placed on the head can be very soothing at the beginning of any style of treatment whether it be massage, acupuncture, shiatsu or aromatherapy and hands resting on the feet at the close of the treatment can add an element of deep relaxation to the treatment.

Naturally, the intent of the Reiki practitioner is different to that of a massage therapist and this will also ensure that the experiences are also quite different. A Reiki practitioner holds the intent to allow healing to take place while a therapist technically works at removing or working with specific physical issues. A massage is far more physical in nature than a Reiki treatment. A Reiki treatment is a spiritually based healing system with the practitioner also constantly working on herself to improve her spiritual connection and inner balance.

A professional Reiki practitioner may not include massage in her treatment without the appropriate qualifications. A practitioner must also be insured for any manipulative techniques that she uses. Here, massage and Reiki also differ as Reiki has no contraindications, unlike massage.

REIKI AND RELIGION

Reiki is available for everyone. It excludes no-one; no matter what age, ethnicity or religious belief. The system of Reiki does not ask for any specific religious affiliation or belief, therefore it is also not necessary to belong to a particular belief system to experience a Reiki treatment.

The simplicity of the fundamental concept of the system makes it suitable to fit within the boundaries of any individual's personal belief system whether the person is a Buddhist, Catholic, Protestant, Muslim, atheist or a member of any other religious or spiritual group.

This basic concept that everything is energy lies at the base of the system of Reiki. Humans are working at becoming whole, becoming One with the energy, when they work with Reiki. This brings them into a state of balance with the universe. Most religions would accept that the more balanced its parishioners, the easier it is for them to be able to practice their faith successfully.

In this way, Reiki can be welcomed as a resource and support for Reiki clients and practitioners to help them with their religious practices. A number of Christian nuns, priests and ministers actually practice the system of Reiki with their parishioners as a healing ministry. Reverend Dawn Van Eyk, a minister in the United Church of Canada and a Reiki teacher, teaches Reiki to the teenagers in her congregation as a "cool" way to help them deal with the changes happening in their lives. Her congregation also reaches out with Reiki treatments to the community. Also in Canada, Sister Eileen Curteis, a Catholic nun and Reiki teacher, teaches Reiki to those who wish to learn it with a strong Christian and spiritual understanding. Many religions have within their own teachings the concept of helping others and self-healing. Many believe the following quote by Jesus relates to humanity's innate healing ability.

Jesus said ...

//

Most assuredly, I say to you, he who believes in Me, the works that I do he will do also; and greater works than these he will do ...

//

Bible (New King James Version): John 14:12-14

If you are concerned that receiving a Reiki treatment may clash with your belief system, a suggestion is to try to find a practitioner from your religious background. This person will most likely be sensitive to your concerns and help to inform you about Reiki in relation to your religion. Attending a Reiki session with uncertainty, especially fear, will only work against the healing effect of your Reiki treatment.

The system of Reiki was developed by a Japanese Buddhist practitioner, Usui Mikao, however, it is understood that he intentionally left out all references to Buddhist practices and deities to make the system accessible to people of all religions.

When you respond to a Reiki treatment you may find yourself connecting with your own religious and/or spiritual beliefs. You may see or feel the presence of a religious being that you relate to. It is understood within the system of Reiki that individuals will translate an energetic or spiritual experience according to their own beliefs.

Heaven on Earth

While Emily, a devout Christian, was lying on the treatment table during her Reiki treatment she experienced some interesting visions. It occurred as she lay on her stomach and the practitioner held her hands at the back of her chest area. Suddenly, Emily felt overwhelmed by a sense of peace and a great white light came toward her, engulfing her completely. Tears streamed down her face, not from pain or discomfort but from inner joy. She felt she was experiencing Heaven on Earth. Afterwards she described it as if she had received a message from God.

The Comforting Presence of Gods

Deepa, a Hindu, was born in Delhi but had recently emigrated. She booked a Reiki treatment to help relieve the stress she was under adapting to her new homeland. During the treatment, while her eyes were shut, she saw a vision of herself on the treatment table with Hindu Deities moving around her, trying to comfort her. What surprised Deepa most was that her Reiki practitioner had no knowledge of Hinduism.

REIKI AND PSYCHIC READINGS

Receiving a Reiki treatment is not the same as visiting a psychic. Though there are many differences, there is also the possibility of some similarities. This will depend upon who your Reiki practitioner or psychic is. A professional Reiki practitioner does not purport to diagnose. She is there to create a space in which you can self-heal utilizing her skills as a professional and a Reiki practitioner. The treatment can occur without a word and still be totally effective. The surface interactions between a client and a Reiki practitioner can create an excellent environment for healing but what it all comes back to is this: you, as the client, must draw on the energy and allow it to work through you to heal and balance. A practitioner, no matter how much advice or interpretation she might offer, cannot heal you. For this reason Reiki practitioners strive to become nothing more than a strong vessel for the energy to move through rather than being an interpretive host for the energy.

Some psychics may work in a similar manner, adding their professionalism to different tools like tarot and angel cards, tea leaves, numerology or energetic communication, while also creating a space where self-healing can take place. A psychic will generally differ from a Reiki practitioner in that she interprets what she sees, hears or intuits and passes this information on to you. This process of interpretation occurs in a human zone, where humans make practical decisions based on their experiences. A psychic, therefore, is an interpretative host for energetic communication, unlike a Reiki practitioner. A client should always keep this in mind when dealing with a psychic and choose one whose interpretative skills are respected and widely acknowledged. In the human zone there is the chance that individual interpretations become clouded by personal values, understandings and judgments.

Working energetically, as a Reiki practitioner does, often means that the practitioner is aware at an energetic level. This does not mean that she is required to interpret the sensations or feelings that she may receive during a treatment for the treatment to be successful. These aspects of a practitioner's experience are not considered to be a part of a Reiki treatment but are rather side-effects caused by an individual's energetic development. Her understanding of this will be relative to her level of experience.

Some Reiki practitioners have been known to indulge in energetic interpretation during a Reiki treatment. This is not considered ethical in a Reiki treatment unless the practitioner has expressly informed the client prior to the treatment that she intends to include an energetic interpretation or diagnosis as an extra method in her Reiki treatment plan. This must be followed up by acceptance of the practice on the client's behalf.

If your Reiki practitioner does begin to tell you all about who she thinks you are, it is best not to get caught up in this energetic rationalization. Instead, take the information with a grain of salt knowing that it is the practitioner's own interpretation (even if it sounds absolutely amazing!).

Some clients attend a Reiki treatment with the desire to receive a Reiki treatment/psychic reading. This may be agreed to by a Reiki practitioner who feels she has the ability to conduct such a treatment. In this situation, as the client's focus for the entire session is on gaining personal insight via interpretation, the client's intent is less aimed at allowing the healing to occur. The focus of the treatment moves from a self-healing experience to that of a psychic reading. It is recommended that if a client is interested in both practices they be experienced separately to gain the most benefit.

Many psychics today recommend that their clients take up Reiki. Perhaps they realize the benefits of promoting self-healing for their clients. It is wonderful and stimulating to hear and experience amazing energetic phenomena but the only person who can heal you is yourself.

REIKI AND SPIRITUAL HEALING

A spiritual experience is one that is not overtly physical. It is something intangible that offers you an experience, which for many, is unrelated to the regular routine of life. It is a connection within and without at the same time, a feeling of oneness with everyone and everything.

Healing means to become whole. Wholeness occurs when all human aspects are brought together into balance with one another. In the flowing river that is you, many elements combine to create your human experience.

Spiritual healing is the coming together of these two elements. Within the system of Reiki these elements are also combined as founding principles of the practice. In fact, Reiki, literally translated, means *spiritual energy* in Japanese – it is that intangible binding energy that moves through you, clearing and, consequently, healing your life and making it whole.

Although the system of Reiki is a spiritual form of healing, this does not directly indicate that it works with the popular notion of spirit guides. The system of Reiki is traditionally a Japanese practice that works with Japanese philosophies and ideals. Spirit guides today are commonly associated with the New Age movement. A spirit guide is not just any spirit, but a spirit that guides and advises. Practitioners working with spirit guides often create from this dimension the concept of beings that are external to themselves. In looking for external help they forget that it is internally where the answers to their spiritual quest reside, waiting to be uncovered.

Remembering a Spiritual Connection

Amanda was a 31-year old mother who, at her first Reiki session, told her practitioner that she felt as if her soul was hurting. After the birth of her daughter she had felt depressed and as if she was gradually loosing her connection with her own inner self; her joy of life and being. The practitioner began her first treatment with the simple intent that Amanda might receive whatever she needed at that moment in her life. After the treatment, Amanda said that she had a feeling that the practitioner had somehow communicated with her soul and she claimed to be feeling much better, already. Amanda received a number of renewing treatments and, finally, joined a Reiki course in order to take even more control of her life and promote deeper healing.

REIKI AND THE NEW AGE MOVEMENT

Since Hawayo Takata's passing in 1980, many New Age techniques and methods have been introduced into the system of Reiki. These techniques include chakras, ceremonial rites, ritual tools, crystals, psychic healing, and other popularized ancient knowledge. There are a number of thoughts as to why New Age variances have filtered into the system of Reiki.

One reason may be that the New Age Movement itself was very exciting in the 1980s. At this time it was at a peak in its popularity and was weaving its way into the psyche of the mainstream. Westerners were discovering the value and beauty of mystical teachings from countries like Egypt and India and the magical teachings of the Native American Indians. Reiki, too, was exciting and felt new in the West and ripe to explode around the world. Some Reiki practitioners were drawn to the concept of a hands-on healing technique that included the razzle dazzle of a variety of New Age techniques and brought the two together.

Another reason for the introduction of New Age practices into the system of Reiki might have been due to the lack of infrastructure that existed after Hawayo Takata's death. Her charismatic presence and experiential and historical knowledge was missed. There was dissension regarding who should continue as the head of Hawayo Takata's teachings. Schisms occurred within the Reiki community. These cracks allowed new practices to be introduced to the system by various Reiki teachers under differing auspices, with a few claiming to have the only true teachings.

And lastly, New Age practices may have swept through the system of Reiki during the 1980s and 90s due to the lack of cultural foundation experienced within the system. Reiki is Japanese in origin and yet most of its Japanese qualities were removed from the system when Hawayo Takata brought it to the West at the beginning of the Second World War. It is understandable that a Japanese practice would not have been acceptable in the US at that time.

Reiki in the West

///

On many occasions while John was her student, Takata said, "I have simplified the system."

///

Hand to Hand
John Harvey Grey

Perhaps, due to this simplification, some practitioners felt there was something missing from the system they were practicing and by including New Age techniques believed they were filling in the "gaps" with interesting practices from other cultures. Fortunately, today there is a general interest in researching the system as a whole Japanese form and art and this is available for Reiki practitioners to experience and study.

A Reiki practitioner who is involved with New Age practices may perform some of these practices during a Reiki treatment: fluffing up your energy field with a feather or other object, placing a singing bowl on your body to resonate, or maybe even gathering information from what she may call her *guides*. None of these elements are traditionally a part of a Reiki treatment and yet may be included by some practitioners. These practices are not harmful in nature unless the practitioner begins to try to manipulate, judge or behave unethically using them. Make sure you enquire as to what the practitioner considers to be a Reiki treatment prior to booking in, in order to make sure that you are fully informed and receiving the treatment that you expect to receive.

RESEARCH INTO REIKI

There is a growing interest in complementary and alternative medicine (CAM) world-wide. Contemporary society is willing to welcome CAM into the mainstream on one proviso – that the systems covered by this umbrella term prove themselves to be at the same standard, and of an even higher standard in some cases, than that of the currently popular conventional western medicine. This condition has caused difficulties for the more esoteric therapies such as Reiki.

The Status of CAM Research

Very little high-quality CAM research exists; reasons for this may include: a lack of training in the principles and methods of research; inadequate research funding and a poor research infrastructure within the CAM sector. Another contributing factor may be methodological issues, with many CAM practitioners believing that conventional research methods are not suitable tools with which to investigate CAM.

House of Lords Select Committee on Science and Technology Report

The UK government consequently offered more research funding to certain CAM sectors. In 2006 in the US, the National Center for CAM (NCCAM) received $122.7 million from Congress to fund research. This new scientific approach to CAM aims to ensure that many more therapies will be accessible in hospital environments and receive a greater respect from, and collaboration with, other health care workers.

Barriers to Reiki in Hospitals

Barriers to CAM adoption in hospitals exist despite the vast and rising interest in this field, CAM remains untapped by hospitals. Three barriers prevent CAM

implementation in hospitals: (1) lack of CAM research and data, (2) reimbursement complexity, and (3) conventional conflict among physician providers.

///

Executive Summary from Journal of Healthcare Management.
Coleen F. Santa Ana

These three issues don't even touch on the major problem: testing the efficacy of Reiki using a conventional Western medical structure. NCCAM lists Reiki as a biofield therapy and states that such therapies have defied measurement to date by reproducible methods. Rigorous scientific research requires the ability to replicate study results. Often with Reiki treatments, the success of the result lies not with the Reiki practitioner but with the client. A practitioner can therefore not replicate a treatment. Science also requires the use of double-blind studies where the participants and researchers are unaware of who belongs to the control or experimental group. Biofield therapies have inherent issues with these requirements.

One pilot study taught a group of research participants the basics of the system of Reiki with only half receiving an attunement; they then performed hands-on healing on stroke patients. The practitioners could not determine which group they belonged to through their energetic sensations and some of the non-Reiki practitioners felt more energetically than those who had received attunements.[32] Sensations experienced during a Reiki treatment are not considered indicative of the level of healing taking place. The study found there was no way to gauge the system's efficacy through its results. This research also failed for not taking into consideration the body's natural programming to heal itself and support healing in others. If the client and practitioner's intent is strong enough, then energy will be offered by the practitioner and drawn on by the client. The practitioner, however, is not required to have studied Reiki for this to occur, it is innate – it is how a mother supports her baby. This natural phenomenon lies at the foundation of the system of Reiki, and becomes a skill that you learn to develop when you study the system in its entirety.

UNACCEPTABLE RESEARCH

To enable the system of Reiki to enter this new era of integrative medicine, research is required. With more funds available, serious scientific research is occurring – but at what cost?

Since 1961 studies dedicated to uncovering the efficacy of biofield therapies have been using live animals in their trials.[33] Using animals to scientifically research the system of Reiki means far more than some animals receiving Reiki while others do not. The truth is that "animal models" are either injected with life threatening illnesses or subjected to suffering that humans would find unacceptable for themselves. The results from the inhumane studies mentioned in this chapter will not be included in *Your Reiki Treatment* due to the methods used to achieve them.

What happens to these animals once the studies are finished? According to The Humane Society: A majority of the animals used in experiments are euthanized (killed) during or after the experiment. In some cases, animals are not euthanized, but die as a result of the research for which they were used.

Using animals to test if Reiki treatments (or the lack thereof) will cause pain, illness or eventual cruel death is against every principle of Reiki. That such acts are performed in the name of Reiki is abhorrent. Does testing the efficacy of Reiki warrant taking the life of, or causing suffering to, an animal?

One Study into Reiki funded by NCCAM described itself thus:

A group of four rats simultaneously received daily noise and Reiki, while two other groups received "sham" Reiki or noise alone. A fourth group did not receive noise or additional treatment. The experiment was performed three times to test for reproducibility.

The result for the rats would be measured thus:

In the rat, stress from noise damages the mesenteric microvasculature, leading to leakage of plasma into the surrounding tissue.[34]

Another research study injected mice with mammary cancers. Some were treated with hands-on-healing while others were simply left to see what would happen to them. This study devastatingly concluded that: Future work should involve testing on various diseases and conventional immunological studies of treatment effects on experimental animals.[35]

These actions are an example of the lack of connectedness, of Oneness with life, which our world is experiencing. Candace B. Pert, a scientist who could not stomach dissecting a frog at school, admitted to finding herself so swept along with the "raw ambition" that permeated her work environment in scientific research that she tried to assuage her guilty conscience with this statement:

Mistreating Animals

///

These white rats had been bred for research, and scientists use them in ways I consider appropriate. In my career, I have never seen animals mistreated or killed in ways that promoted suffering."

///

Molecules of Emotion
Candace B. Pert Ph.D.

The words "mistreated" and "suffering" must be relative to one's personal definition but surely deliberately hurting or killing an animal in any way is a form of mistreatment. That one animal, according to scientists, has less right to a life of love and care without pain or disease than another is illogical. That these actions could ever take place in the name of Reiki is unthinkable.

Is the Reiki community willing to forgo its founding spiritual principles to find easier acceptance within conventional western medicine? This in effect would destroy the system of Reiki by pulling its foundation out from underneath it. Perhaps the Reiki community can help create change by shining a bright light on medical research and teaching the important principles of compassion and equal respect for all living things.

There must be an immediate stop to the maiming and killing of animals simply to prove that Reiki works.

FINDING SUPPORTIVE COMMUNITIES

If the concept and principles of the system of Reiki are of interest to you, you may wish to become involved with other like-minded groups in your community.

The system of Reiki, as a holistic system, believes that everything you do in your life affects its quality; every thought, every action and every choice is important. Therefore, like-minded groups are ones that do not focus on material gain but rather foster self-development, the growth of inner knowledge, compassion for the self and others and a strong sense of connection with one's environment.

Energetic and physical practices such as yoga or qi gong are excellent for both mind and body as an additional weekly practice. You will find these classes in much the same way you would find a Reiki treatment, either through word-of-mouth, magazines, or bulletin boards listed in community centers.

Other weekly classes that you may wish to attend are meditation classes. These can be run by a number of spiritual groups and religions including Christian churches, Buddhist centers, Baha'i temples and spiritually oriented community centers.

After your Reiki treatment you may wish to talk to someone about your treatment. This can be difficult if none of your family members are interested in Reiki or self-development, or, worse, don't approve of it – which is sometimes the case. Instead of keeping your experiences bottled up make sure you contact your Reiki practitioner to discuss what is going on and support will be offered you. Some clients may expect that a practitioner rings them as a follow-up to their treatment. This is most unlikely to occur and, in fact, it should not be encouraged as your Reiki treatment is about your healing and you must be proactive in its execution.

Online Reiki forums also exist for those interested in Reiki and who enjoy chatting on the internet with others. However, you can never be 100% sure who is at the other end of an email, so caution is advised. It may also be extremely confusing to your understanding of Reiki to listen to some of the New Age concepts that abound.

A natural follow-on from a Reiki treatment is to complete a Reiki course where, if you choose your course wisely, you will find yourself in a supportive community with ongoing activities.

Communicating with Others about Your Treatment

It can be difficult to discuss with others what you experienced during your Reiki treatment. Here are some ways of opening up positive communication with family and friends about it. Being able to discuss your treatment can be very empowering.

I experienced a Japanese relaxation treatment called Reiki. It works at balancing out the mind, body and spirit. It was very gentle and non-invasive and afterward I felt (perhaps one of the following is helpful):

• Calm and peaceful.

• Clear.

• Renewed.

• Inspired.

Reiki treatments today are available everywhere. You can experience them in health spas, hospitals, Medical Centers or at your local natural therapy center.

Extra Tip: You could even give a family member a Reiki treatment gift voucher. An experience is often stronger than the spoken word.

Moving on to a Reiki Course

Taking your Power

///

*We cannot live in a world that is not our own, in a world that is interpreted
for us by others. An interpreted world is not a home. Part of the terror is to
take back our own listening, to use our own voice, to see our own light.*

///

Hildegard Von Bingen

Your Reiki treatment experience has piqued your curiosity to find out
more about how you can become more proactive in healing yourself;
wanting to live a fulfilled life is a natural human characteristic.

If you would like to take your Reiki treatment up a notch into a
realm of personal empowerment then perhaps a Reiki course is for
you.

In a Level I course, with a teacher to guide and support you, you
will learn how to help yourself, friends and family. There are a
number of critical elements to a Level I course which you will need
to study. Usui Mikao utilized these traditional elements to bring
about an unmasking, a revelation of what it meant to be human.
From this perspective you will find that it is not the energy that is
unique in the system of Reiki but the path that is walked.

There are various styles of Reiki courses. Below are the fundamental elements that you will experience in a Reiki course when
taught from a traditional Japanese perspective.

Precepts

The five precepts of Reiki create the foundation of the system of
Reiki. Each of the other elements were formed with these precepts
at their heart. Translated from the Japanese word gokai.

Reiki Techniques and Meditations

These practices aid you in sensing your connection to energy,
grounding yourself in life, and gaining a broader perspective on

the human experience. The more you practice these techniques, the more energy you will be able to move in your body to help yourself and others. Meditation is recognized as an antidote to stress, an aid to clarity of thought and a wonderful relaxant.

Hands-on healing

Working with your hands is a gentle way to discover the joys of spiritual practice. You learn how to place your hands on the body, offering energy to it, supporting the body with its natural cleansing process. Hands-on healing gradually brings you into a deeper connection with universal energy, your home. Translated from the Japanese words tenohira and teate.

Symbols and mantras

These tools teach you the interrelationship between certain aspects of universal energy. This element is only taught in Level II and III of the system of Reiki as you experientially delve deeper into its meanings. Translated from the Japanese words shirushi and jumon.

Spiritual Blessing

The last major element of the system of Reiki is the receiving of reiju, or spiritual blessing, from a teacher (reiju is a blessing from which the Western attunement evolved).

The first four elements become part of a personal daily routine and, if possible, should be coupled with the regular receiving of reiju. When brought together each of the elements exerts a separate influence on the practitioner producing a complete system that affects powerful change.

This spiritual teaching is accessible to everyone. Each element supports the other, filling in the gaps that will exist for different practitioners. No two people have the same needs when learning. For this reason working with all elements gives each practitioner a greater chance of success in finding that inner home.

SUPPORT TOOLS

Tools are resources for developing a better theoretical understanding of your therapy and for stimulating a deeper experiential understanding of your practice.

Here are a couple of recommended tools that will help you delve further into the system of Reiki. These products include books, cards, CDs and even an online program. It is not necessary to have studied the system of Reiki to be able to enjoy any of these Reiki products.

The Japanese Art of Reiki

This is a book that looks solely at the Japanese self-healing aspects of the system of Reiki and guides you through them. All branches of Reiki have at their foundation five basic elements. Step-by-step you are taken on a journey of self-healing using these elements including traditional meditations and techniques, precepts and hands-on healing. Learn about each element and how to use it from its traditional Japanese perspective guided by the fully illustrated text.

The Reiki Sourcebook and A-Z of Reiki Pocketbook

These two books will teach you everything you need to know about Reiki from when it first began to the multitude of ideas that exist about it today. You can go pocket-sized with the *A-Z of Reiki Pocketbook* or you can get the whole story with the weighty *The Reiki Sourcebook*.

Reiki Techniques Card Deck

You do not need to be a Reiki practitioner to benefit from this unusual healing card deck. Everyone on the planet has the ability to initiate self-healing – it is your birthright. The techniques in this deck of 45 cards, selected from the most effective traditional and non-traditional Reiki techniques from around the globe, offer you the opportunity to consciously tap into your healing ability, supporting you on your natural path.

Guided Meditation CDs

Reiki Tenohira CD
A guided practice of the Reiki hand positions for self-healing with meditation music. Includes a fold-out booklet with illustrations.

Reiki Hô
A guided practice of the traditional Japanese Reiki technique Hatsurei Hô with Japanese-inspired meditation music, designed to strengthen your hara. Includes a fold-out booklet with illustrations.

Reiki Kan
Music for intuitive Reiki treatments and meditation. Kan is a Japanese word that refers to learning through direct experience, personal discovery and intuition. This is one continuous 60-minute track.

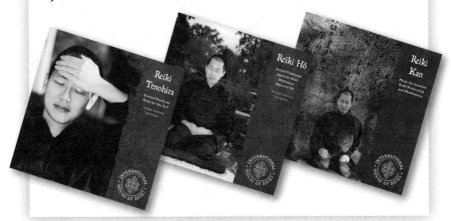

Online 21-Day Reiki Program

Sign up online at *www.reiki.net.au* and each day, for 21 days, you receive an email that guides you on a journey of self-healing. An intense period that uses elements of the system of Reiki to initiate clearing in the body, support you in developing a regular routine and teach you about the practices from a Japanese influenced perspective. Apart from a traditional Reiki approach to clearing there are also suggestions and directions from various cultures to broaden your understanding of the process you are undertaking. In this manner you will also begin to see that clearing is a natural part of the human existence.

Online
21-Day
Reiki Program

Glossary

Biofield Therapy – Therapies listed under CAM that are believed to act by correcting imbalances in the internal biofield, such as by restoring the flow of qi through meridians to reinstate health. Some therapists are believed to emit or transmit the vital energy (external qi) to a recipient to restore health. (Definition according to NCCAM)

CAM – A broad domain of healing resources that encompasses all health systems, modalities, and practices and their accompanying theories and beliefs, other than those intrinsic to the politically dominant health systems of a particular society or culture in a given historical period. (Definition according to the UK Department of Health)

Distant Healing – This method is used to send Reiki to someone who is not physically present.

Duty of Care – A practitioner's responsibility to the client.

Enlightenment – An enlightened state is one where there is a unique awareness of existence; to hold an understanding of the perfection of yourself within the perfection of the universe and to act in accordance with that.

Hara – According to Japanese energetic practices, the hara is a major energy center in the body which can be experienced in the belly or abdomen.

Level I – The first level of training in a Reiki course.

Level II – The second level of training in a Reiki course.

Level III – The final level of training in a Reiki course.

NCCAM – National Center for Complementary and Alternative Medicine.

Okuden – The Japanese name for the second level of training in a Reiki course.

Reiki – Translated from the Japanese to mean *spiritual energy* and is also known in the West as universal life force energy.

Reiki, the system of – A system started in the early 1900s by Usui Mikao in Japan. It consists of five main elements: precepts, meditations and techniques, hands-on healing, symbols and mantras and attunements or reiju. Traditionally it has three levels and is taught as a spiritual practice which encompasses self-healing and the ability to heal others.

Reiki Master – The label given to a Reiki student who has completed all three levels of Reiki including how to perform an attunement or reiju. It does not mean that this person has mastered Reiki or that this person has received specific teacher training. A Reiki Master may also go by the name of Reiki Teacher or Reiki Master/ Teacher or have completed Shinpiden.

Reiki Practitioner – A person who has completed at least the first level of a Reiki course.

Reiki Precepts – The precepts are the Reiki practitioner's first spiritual teachings and are universal and open to anyone regardless of their personal religious beliefs. They are:

For today only:

Do not anger

Do not worry

Be humble

Be honest in your work

Be compassionate to yourself and others

Reiki Ryôhô Hikkei – A manual put together by the Usui Reiki Ryôhô Gakkai for its members.

Reiki Session – Includes all aspects of a Reiki treatment that are contained within your Reiki appointment timeslot.

Reiki Teacher – The label given to a Reiki student who has completed all three levels of Reiki including how to perform an attunement or reiju. It does not mean that this person has mastered Reiki or that this person has received specific teacher training. A Reiki Teacher may also go by the name of Reiki Master or Reiki Master/Teacher or have completed Shinpiden.

Reiki Treatment – Includes the actual treatment where a practitioner places hands on, or near, the body while the client draws on the energy.

Primary Health Care – This was a new approach to health care that came into existence following an international conference in Alma Ata in 1978 organized by the World Health Organization and UNICEF. Primary health care is defined as follows: Primary health care is essential health care based on practical, scientifically sound and socially acceptable methods and technology made universally accessible to individuals and families in the community through their full participation and at a cost that the community and the country can afford to maintain at every stage of their development in the spirit of self-determination.

Shinpiden – The Japanese name for the third level of a Reiki course. See Reiki Teacher.

Shoden – The second level of training in a Reiki course.

Notes

1 Physicians Attitudes toward CAM and their Knowledge of Specific Therapies: A Survey at an Academic Medical Center. eCam. 2006, USA. Dietlind L. Wahner-Roedler, Ann Vincent, Peter L. Elkin, Laura L. Loehrer, Stephen S. Cha and Brent A. Bauer.

2 Physicians Attitudes toward CAM and their Knowledge of Specific Therapies: A Survey at an Academic Medical Center. eCam. 2006, USA. Dietlind L. Wahner-Roedler, Ann Vincent, Peter L. Elkin, Laura L. Loehrer, Stephen S. Cha and Brent A. Bauer.

3 Oschman, James L. Energy Medicine – The Scientific Basis, Churchill Livingstone, London, 2000.

4 In Vitro Effect of Reiki Treatment on Bacterial Cultures: Role of Experimental Context and Practitioner WellBeing. Journal of Alternative and Complementary Medicine. 2006, January. Vol. 12. No. 1: 7-13. Beverly Rubik, Ph.D., Audrey J. Brooks, Ph.D., Gary E. Schwartz, Ph.D.

5 Reiki Ryôhô Hikkei, manual from the Usui Reiki Ryôhô Gakkai, Japan.

6 Weir, Michael. Complementary Medicine – Ethics and Law, Prometheus Publications, Brisbane, 2000.

7 Surgeon General's report on Mental Health, 1999, USA.

8 See Glossary for a full copy of the Reiki Precepts.

9 Diagnosis Cancer: The Science & Controversy Behind Touch Therapies Patients claim benefit, but some doctors question evidence. Cure. Spring Issue 2005. Jennifer M. Gangloff.

10 Patient Care Report. 2004. Brownes Cancer Support Centre.

11 Oschman, James L. Energy Medicine – The Scientific Basis, Churchill Livingstone, London, 2000.

12   Oschman, James L. Energy Medicine – The Scientific Basis, Churchill Livingstone, London, 2000.

13   Oschman, James L. Energy Medicine – The Scientific Basis, Churchill Livingstone, London, 2000.

14   Diagnosis Cancer: The Science & Controversy Behind Touch Therapies Cure. Spring Issue 2005. Jennifer M. Gangloff.

15   Attitudes In The American Workplace VI Gallup Poll sponsored by the Marlin Company, 2000.

16   Attitudes In The American Workplace VI Gallup Poll sponsored by the Marlin Company, 2000.

17   Attitudes In The American Workplace VI Gallup Poll sponsored by the Marlin Company, 2000.

18   National Institute of Mental Health. USA.

19   National Institute of Mental Health. USA.

20   Long-term Effects of Energetic Healing on Symptoms of Psychological Depression and Self-perceived Stress. Alternative Therapies Health and Medicine. 2004, Vol. 10. Issue 3, Pages 42-48. A. G. Shore.

21   Neutralizing Workplace Stress: The Physiology of Human Performance and Organizational Effectiveness. Presented at: Psychological Disabilities in the Workplace at the Center for Professional Learning. 1996, June 12. Toronto, Canada. Bruce A. Cryer.

22   The Use of Reiki in Psychotherapy. Perspectives in Psychiatric Care. 2005, October. 41 (4). 184-187. Mary Ann LaTorre.

23   UCLA Neuropsychiatric Institute.

24   Deconstructing the Placebo Effect and Finding the Meaning Response. Annals of Internal Medicine 2002, 19 March. Volume 136 Issue 6, Pages 471-476. Daniel E. Moerman, PhD. and Wayne B. Jonas, MD.

25   Analgesic Effects of Branding in Treatment of Headaches. British Medical Journal (Clin. Res. Ed.) 1981, May 16. 282(6276): 1576–1578. A. Branthwaite and P. Cooper.

26   Deconstructing the Placebo Effect and Finding the Meaning Response. Annals of Internal Medicine 2002, 19 March. Volume 136 Issue 6, Pages 471-476. Daniel E. Moerman, PhD. and Wayne B. Jonas, MD.

27 Weir, Michael. Complementary Medicine – Ethics and Law, Prometheus Publications, Brisbane, 2000.

28 Role of Fever in Disease. Annals of the New York Academy of Sciences. 1998, September. Vol. 856 Page 224. Matthew J. Kluger, Wieslaw Kozak, Carole A. Conn, Lisa R. Leon, Dariusz Soszynski

29 Reiki Ryôhô Hikkei, manuals from the Usui Reiki Ryôhô Gakkai, Japan.

30 According to Transcendental Meditation research.

31 Evaluation of Healing by Gentle Touch in 35 Patients with Cancer. European Journal of Oncology Nursing. 2004, 8, 40-49. C Weze, HL Leathard, J Grange, P Tiplady, & G Stevens.

32 Effect of Reiki Treatments on Functional Recovery in Patients in Poststroke Rehabilitation: a Pilot Study. Journal of Alternative and Complementary Medicine. 2002 December. SC Shiflett, S Nayak, C Bid, P Miles, S Agostinelli.

33 The Influence of an Unorthodox Method of Treatment on Wound Healing in Mice. International Journal of Parapsychology. 1961. 3, p. 5-24. B. Grad, R.J. Cadoret, G.I. Paul.

34 Personal Interaction with a Reiki Practitioner Decreases Noise-Induced Microvascular Damage in an Animal Model. Journal of Alternative and Complementary Medicine. 2006, January. Vol. 12. No. 1: 15-22. Ann L. Baldwin Ph.D., Gary E. Schwartz.

35 The Effect of the "Laying On of Hands" on Transplanted Breast Cancer in Mice. Journal of Scientific Exploration. 2000, Volume 14: Number 3: Article 2. William F. Bengston and David Krinsley.

Bibliography

Arnold, Larry and Sandy Nevius. The Reiki Handbook, Psi, Oregon, 1992.

Barnett, Libby. *Reiki Energy Medicine: Bringing the Healing Touch into Home, Hospital and Hospice*, Healing Arts Press, Vermont, 1996.

Bary De, WM Theodore. *Sources of Japanese Tradition*, Columbian University Press, New York, 2001.

Blacker, Carmen. *The Catalpa Bow – A Study of Shamanic Practices in Japan*, Japan Library, Richmond, 1999.

Breen, John and Mark Teeuwen. *Shinto in History – Ways of the Kami*, Curzon Press, Surrey, 2000.

Brown, Fran. *Living Reiki – Takata's Teachings*, Life Rhythm, California, 1992.

Buxton-King, Angie. *The NHS Healer*, Virgin Books, London, 2004.

Cleary, Thomas. *The Japanese Art of War – Understanding the Culture of Strategy*, Shambhala Publications, Boston, 1991.

Cohen, Kenneth S. *The Way of QiGong*, Ballantine Books, New York, 1997.

Curteis, Eileen. *Reiki – A Spiritual Doorway To Natural Healing*, Lightning Source Inc, La Vergne, 2004.

Davey, H.E. *Japanese Yoga – The Way of Dynamic Meditation*, Stone Bridge Press, Berkeley, 2001.

Davey, H.E. *Living the Japanese Arts & Ways*, Stone Bridge Press, Berkeley, 2003.

Doi, Hiroshi. *Modern Reiki Method for Healing*, Fraser Journal Publishing, British Columbia, 2000.

Ellis, Richard. *Practical Reiki – Focus Your Body's Energy for Deep Relaxation and Inner Peace*, Sterling Publishing Company, New York, 1999.

Floyd, H. Ross. *Shintô – The Way of Japan*, Greenwood Publishing

Group, Westport, 1965.

Funakoshi, Gichin. *Karate-dô – My Way of Life*, Kodansha America Inc, New York, 1975.

Gleinsner, Earlene F. *Reiki in Everyday Living*, Jaico Publishing House, Delhi, 1997.

Gordon, Andrew. *A Modern History of Japan – From Tokugawa Times to the Present*, Oxford University Press, Oxford, 2002.

Gray, John Harvey and Lourdes. *Hand to Hand – The Longest-Practicing Reiki Master Tells His Story*, Xlibris Corporation, 2002.

Green, Brian. *The Fabric of the Cosmos – Space, Time, and the Texture of Reality*, Vintage, London, 2005.

Groner, Paul. *Saicho – The Establishment of the Japanese Tendai School*, University of Hawaii Press, Honolulu, 2000.

Gyatso, Tenzin. (Dalai Lama) *Kindness, Clarity and Insight*, Wisdom Publications, New York, 1984.

Haberly, Helen J. *Reiki – Hawayo Takata's Story*, Archedigm Publications, Maryland, 2000.

Hall, Mari. *Practical Reiki – A Practical Step by Step Guide to this Ancient Healing Art*, Thorsons, London, 1997.

Hall, Mari. *Reiki for Common Ailments – A Practical Guide to Healing*, Piatkus, London, 1999.

Hanh, Thich Nhat. *Opening the Heart of the Cosmos – Insights on the Lotus Sutra*, Paralax Press, Berkeley, 2003.

Hanh, Thich Nhat. *The Diamond that Cuts Through Illusion – Commentaries on the Prajnaparamita Diamond Sutra*, Paralax Press, Berkeley, 1992.

Hayashi, Chûjirô. *Ryôhô Shishin*, Japan.

Hitoshi, Miyake. *Shugendô – Essays on the Structure of Japanese Folk Religion*, The University of Michigan, Michigan, 2001.

Honervogt, Tanmaya. *The Power of Reiki – An Ancient Hands-On Healing System*, Henry Holt and Company, Inc, New York, 1998.

Horan, Paula. *Abundance Through Reiki*, Windpferd, Aitrang, 1990.

Horan, Paula. *Exploring Reiki – 108 Questions & Answers*, New Page Books, New York, 2005.

Humphrey, Nicholas. *The Mind Made Flesh*, Oxford University Press, 2002.

Inagaki, Hisao. *A Dictionary of Japanese Buddhist Terms*, Nagata Bunshodo, Kyoto, 2003.

Jahnke, Roger. *The Healing Promise of Qi*, Contemporary Books, New York, 2002.

Keene, Donald. *Emperor of Japan – Meiji and His World, 1852-1912*, Columbia University Press, New York, 2002.

Kelly, Maureen J. *Reiki and the Healing Buddha*, Lotus Press, Twin Lakes, 2000.

Lubeck, Walter. *The Complete Reiki Handbook*, Windpferd, Aitrang, 1990.

Lubeck, Walter., Frank Arjava Petter and William Lee Rand. *The Spirit of Reiki*, Lotus Press, Twin Lakes, 2001.

Lugenbeel, Barbara. *Virginia Samdahl – Reiki Master Healer*, Grunwald and Radcliff, 1984.

Mendizza, Michael., and Joseph Chilton Pearce. *Magical Parent-Magical Child – The Optimum Learning Relationship*, North Atlantic Books, Berkeley, 2004.

Mihashi Kazuo. *Tenohira-ga Byoki-o Naosu*, Chuo Art Publishing Co., Ltd., 2001.

Mitchell, Paul David. *Reiki – The Usui System of Natural Healing (The Blue Book)*, Mitchel, Paul David, Idaho, 1985.

Mizutani, Osamu and Nobuku. *An Introduction to Modern Japanese*, Japan Times Ltd, Tôkyô, 1977.

Mochizuki, Toshitaka. *Iyashi No Te*, Tama Shuppan, Tôkyô, 1995.

Mochizuki, Toshitaka. *Chô Kantan Iyashi No Te*, Tama Shuppan, Tôkyô, 2001.

Motz, Julie. *Hands of Life*, Bantam Books, 1998.

Nishida, Tenko. *A New Road to Ancient Truth*, Horizon Press, New York, 1972.

Oda, Ryuko. *Kaji-Empowerment and Healing in Esoteric Buddhism*, Kineizan Shinjao-in Mitsumonkai, Japan, 1992.

Oschman, James L. *Energy Medicine – The Scientific Basis*, Churchill Livingstone, London, 2000.

Paramhans Swami Maheshwarananda. *The Hidden Power in Humans*, Ibera Verlag, Vienna, 2004.

Pearce, Joseph Chilton. *The Biology Of Transcendence – A Blueprint of the Human Spirit*, Park Street Press, Vermont, 2004.

Pert, Candace B. *Molecules of Emotion – Why You Feel The Way You Feel*, Simon & Schuster Uk Ltd, London, 1997.

Petter, Frank Arjava. *The Original Reiki Handbook of Dr. Mikao Usui*, Lotus Press, Twin Lakes, 1999.

Prasad, Kathleen, Elizabeth Fulton. *Animal Reiki – Using Energy to Heal the Animals in Your Life*, Ulysses Press, Berkeley, 2006.

Radha, Swami Sivananda. *Kundalini Yoga for the West*, Shambhala Publications, Boston, 1981.

Rand, William Lee. *Reiki – The Healing Touch*, Vision Publications, Michigan, 2000.

Reader, Ian. *Religion in Contemporary Japan*, University of Hawaii Press, Hawaii, 1991.

Reed, William. *Ki – A Practical Guide for Westerners*, Japan Publications Inc, Tôkyô, 1986.

Reiki Ryôhô Hikkei, Usui Reiki Ryôhô Gakkai, Japan.

Sargent, Jiho. *Asking About Zen – 108 Answers*, Weatherhill, Inc. New York, 2001.

Steven, John. *Sacred Calligraphy of the East*, Shambhala Publications, Boston, 1996.

Steven, John. *The Marathon Monks of Mount Hiei*, Shambhala Publications, Boston 1988.

Stiene, Bronwen and Frans. *A-Z of Reiki Pocketbook – Everything About Reiki*, O Books, Winchester, 2006.

Stiene, Bronwen and Frans. *Reiki Techniques Card Deck – Heal Yourself Intuitively*, O Books, Winchester, 2006.

Stiene, Bronwen and Frans. *The Japanese Art of Reiki*, O Books, Winchester, 2005.

Stiene, Bronwen and Frans. *The Reiki Sourcebook*, O Books, Winchester, 2003.

Suzuki, D.T. *Buddha of Infinite Light – The Teachings of Shin Buddhism, The Japanese Way of Wisdom and Compasion*, Shambhala Publications, Boston, 1998.

Suzuki, D.T. *Manual of Zen Buddhism*, Rider & Company, London, 1986.

Suzuki, Shunryu. *Zen Mind, Beginners Mind*, Weatherhill, New York, 1970.

Suzuki, Shunryu. *Branching Streams Flow in the Darkness: Lectures on the Sandokai*, University of California Press, Berkeley, 1999.

Suzuki, Shunryu, *Not Always So – Practicing the True Spirit of Zen*, HarperCollins, New York, 2002.

Takata Furumoto, Alice. *The Gray Book*, Takata Furumoto, Alice, 1982.

Tanabe, George J. Jr. *Religions of Japan in Practice*, Princeton University Press, Princeton, 1999.

Tohei, Koichi. *Ki in Daily Life*, Ki-no-Kenkyûkai, Tôkyô, 1980.

Tohei, Koichi. *Book of Ki – Coordinating Mind and Body in Daily Life*, Japan Publications Inc, Tôkyô, 1976.

Tomita, Kaiji. *Reiki To Jinjutsu – Tomita Ryû Teate Ryôhô*, BAB Japan, Tôkyô, 1999.

Turnbull, Stephen R. *Ninja – The True Story of Japan's Secret Warrior Cult*, Firebird Publishers, Belleville, 1992.

Twan, Anelli. *Early Days of Reiki – Memories of Hawayo Takata*, Morning Star Productions, Hope, 2005.

Twan, Wanja. *In the Light of a Distant Star – A Spiritual Journey Bringing the Unseen into the Seen*, Morning Star Productions, Hope.

Unno, Taitetsu. *River of Fire – River of Water, An Introduction to the Pure Land Tradition of Shin Buddhism*, Doubleday, New York, 1998.

Varley, Paul. *Japanese Culture*, University of Hawaii Press, Honolulu, 2000.

Wangyal, Tenzin. *Healing with Form, Energy and Light*, Snow Lion Publications, Boulder, 2002.

Watson, Burton. *The Lotus Sutra*, Columbia University Press, New York, 1993.

Weir, Michael. *Complementary Medicine – Ethics and Law*, Prometheus Publications, Brisbane, 2000.

Yandrick, Rudy. *Behavioral Risk Management – How to Avoid Preventable Losses from Mental Health Problems in the Workplace*, Jossey-Bass Publishers, San Francisco, 1996.

Yun, Hsing. *Describing the Indescribable*, Wisdom Publications, Boston, 2001.

Journals and Reports:

Alternative Medicines Gain in Popularity, Merit Closer Scrutiny
Journal of the National Cancer Institute
1999, July. Vol. 91, No. 13. pp. 1104-1105.
Katherine Arnold

Analgesic Effects of Branding in Treatment of Headaches
British Medical Journal (Clin. Res. Ed.)
1981, May 16. 282(6276): 1576–1578.
A. Branthwaite and P. Cooper

Attitudes In The American Workplace Report
VI Gallup Poll sponsored by the Marlin Company, 2000.

Autonomic Nervous System Changes During Reiki Treatment: A Preliminary Study
Journal of Alternative and Complementary Medicine
2004, December. Vol. 10. No. 6: 1077-1081.
N. Mackay, S. Hansen, O. McFarlane

Complementary and Alternative Medicine
House of Lords Select Committee on Science and Technology Report
November 2000

Deconstructing the Placebo Effect and Finding the Meaning Response
Annals of Internal Medicine
2002, 19 March. Volume 136 Issue 6, Pages 471-476.
Daniel E. Moerman, PhD. and Wayne B. Jonas, MD

Diagnosis Cancer: The Science & Controversy Behind Touch Therapies
Cure Spring Issue 2005.
Jennifer M. Gangloff

Effect of Reiki Treatments on Functional Recovery in Patients in
Poststroke Rehabilitation: a Pilot Study
Journal of Alternative and Complementary Medicine
2002 December
SC Shiflett, S Nayak, C Bid, P Miles, S Agostinelli

Evaluation of Healing by Gentle Touch in 35 Patients with Cancer
European Journal of Oncology Nursing
2004, 8, 40-49.
C Weze, HL Leathard, J Grange, P Tiplady, & G Stevens

Executive Summary from Journal of Healthcare Management
James Madison University 2001
Coleen F. Santa Ana

In Vitro Effect of Reiki Treatment on Bacterial Cultures: Role of Ex-
perimental Context and Practitioner WellBeing
Journal of Alternative and Complementary Medicine
2006, January. Vol. 12. No. 1: 7-13.
Beverly Rubik, Ph.D., Audrey J. Brooks, Ph.D., Gary E. Schwartz,
Ph.D.

Japanese Journals of Religious Studies
Nanzan Institute for Religion and Culture, Japan.

Long-term Effects of Energetic Healing on Symptoms of Psychological Depression and Self-perceived Stress
Alternative Therapies Health and Medicine
2004, Vol. 10. Issue 3, Pages 42-48.
A. G. Shore

Neutralizing Workplace Stress: The Physiology of Human Perform-
ance and Organizational Effectiveness
Presented at: Psychological Disabilities in the Workplace at the
Center for Professional Learning.
1996, June 12. Toronto, Canada.
Bruce A. Cryer

Patient Care Report.
Brownes Cancer Support Centre
2004, Australia.

Personal Interaction with a Reiki Practitioner Decreases Noise-Induced Microvascular Damage in an Animal Model
Journal of Alternative and Complementary Medicine
2006, January. Vol. 12. No. 1: 15-22.
Ann L. Baldwin Ph.D., Gary E. Schwartz

Physicians Attitudes toward CAM and their Knowledge of Specific Therapies: A Survey at an Academic Medical Center.
eCam
2006, USA.
Dietlind L. Wahner-Roedler, Ann Vincent, Peter L. Elkin, Laura L. Loehrer, Stephen S. Cha and Brent A. Bauer

Role of Fever in Disease
Annals of the New York Academy of Sciences
1998, September. Vol. 856 Page 224.
Matthew J. Kluger, Wieslaw Kozak, Carole A. Conn, Lisa R. Leon, Dariusz Soszynski

Surgeon General's report on Mental Health.
1999, USA.

The Effect of the "Laying On of Hands" on Transplanted Breast Cancer in Mice
Journal of Scientific Exploration
2000, Volume 14: Number 3: Article 2.
William F. Bengston and David Krinsley

The Influence of an Unorthodox Method of Treatment on Wound Healing in Mice
International Journal of Parapsychology
1961. 3, p. 5-24.
B. Grad, R.J. Cadoret, G.I. Paul

The Origins of Human Love and Violence
Pre- and Perinatal Psychology Journal
1996, Spring. Volume 10. Number 3: pp. 143-188.
James W. Prescott, Ph.D.

The Silent Health Care Revolution: The Rising Demand for Complementary Medicine
Nursing Economics
1999, 17, no. 5: 246-53.
L. Strasen

The Use of Reiki in Psychotherapy
Perspectives in Psychiatric Care
2005, October. 41 (4). 184-187.
Mary Ann LaTorre

Index

Remember...

I am open to receive whatever it is that I may need at this exact moment in my life.

Other O-books of interest

The Reiki Sourcebook
BRONWEN AND FRANS STIENE

It captures everything a Reiki practitioner will ever need to know about the ancient art. This book is hailed by most Reiki professionals as the best guide to Reiki. For an average reader, it's also highly enjoyable and a good way to learn to understand Buddhism, therapy and healing. – **Michelle Bakar**, Beauty magazine

9781903816554/1903816556•384pp £12.99 $19.95

A-Z of Reiki Pocketbook
Everything About Reiki
BRONWEN AND FRANS STIENE

A-Z of Reiki, *the latest work by Bronwen and Frans Stiene, is an all-encompassing and expansive glossary of Reiki and Japanese healing. This book helps clear the way for everyone to partake of Reiki.* – **Nina Paul**, author of Reiki for Dummies

9781905047895/1905047894•272pp•125x90mm £7.99 $16.95

Energy Works!
Initiation without a master
TERESA PARROTT AND GRAHAM CROOK

Graham and Teresa have explored the world of SKHM to a depth that few have been able to achieve, and, most importantly, they have been able to share their experience with others through their words in the most beautiful way. Those who read about their experience will be initiated in a journey of the heart. – **Patrick Zeigler**

9781905047529/1905047525•304pp £12.99 $24.95

Healing Hands
Simple and practical reflexology techniques for developing god health and inner peace
DAVID VENNELLS

Promising good health and inner peace, this practical guide to reflexology techniques may not be a glossy affair but it is thoroughly and clearly illustrated. Healing Hands *can support your journey.* – **Wave**

9781905047123/1905047126•192pp £9.99 $16.95

The Japanese Art of Reiki
A practical guide to self healing
BRONWEN AND FRANS STIENE

This is a sequel to the aclaimed "Reiki Sourcebook." For those of us in the West who see adverts for weekend Reiki Master courses and wonder about the authenticity of the tradition, this book is an eye-opener. It takes the reader back to the Japanese roots of the tradition in a way that conveys its inspirational power and cultural flavour.
– **Medical Network Review** 9781905047024/1905047029•208pp £12.99 $19.95

Reiki Jin Kei Do
The way of compassion and wisdom
STEVE GOOCH

Steve Gooch has done an excellent job in presenting to the public the world's first book on the deeply profound and beautiful teachings that were given to me by Seiji Takamori. In doing so he has become the spokesperson for the whole lineage. I recommend it highly to all. – **Dr Ranga Premaratna**, Lineage Head of Reiki Jin Kei Do

9781905047857/1905047851•260pp £12.99 $21.95

Reiki Q&A: 200 Questions & Answers for Beginners
LAWRENCE ELLYARD

This unique handbook clearly answers all kinds of questions about Reiki and its practice as well as dispelling any misconceptions. Useful, dependable and highly recommended. – **Penny Parkes**, author of *15-minute Reiki*

9781905047475/1905047479•208pp £12.99 $24.95

New Reiki Mastery
For second degree students and masters
DAVID VENNELLS

A compassionate, wise, handbook to making the most of the Life Force Energy that surrounds and informs us all. *An excellent reference for anyone interested in hands-on healing. Helpful and insightful, good and solid.* – **Amazon**

9781903816707/190381670X•192pp £9.99 $14.95

Reiki Techniques Card Deck
Heal Yourself Intuitively

BRONWEN AND FRANS STIENE

Everyone has the ability to initiate self-healing-it is your birthright. The techniques in this deck of 45 cards, selected from the most effective traditional and non-traditional Reiki techniques from around the globe, offer you the opportunity to consciously tap into your healing ability, supporting you on your natural path.

9781905047192/1905047193•24pp•40 colour cards•box•88x127mm £15.99 $24.95

Ultimate Reiki Guide for Practitioners and Masters

LAWRENCE ELLYARD

In this excellent volume, Lawrence Ellyard brings together his considerable expertise and experience to provide a clear and concise view of how to conduct Reiki and to establish oneself as a Reiki practitioner. It will be invaluable for all Reiki professionals and lay persons as a spiritual, practice and business guide.
– **Dr. Ralph Locke**, CEO, Ikon

9781905047482/1905047487•208pp £12.99 $24.95

Your Reiki Treatment

BRONWEN AND FRANS STIENE

This is the first title to look at Reiki from the client's perspective. Whether you are searching for relaxation, healing, or spiritual growth, a Reiki treatment can be a revelation. Find out how to make the most of it. Learn how to prepare, what to expect, and how to continue furthering your personal growth after the treatment is finished.

9781846940132/18469490133•240pp £9.99 $19.95

O

is a symbol of the world,
of oneness and unity. O Books
explores the many paths of wholeness and spiritual understanding which
different traditions have developed down
the ages. It aims to bring this knowledge in
accessible form, to a general readership, providing practical spirituality to today's seekers.

For the full list of over 200 titles covering:
ACADEMIC/THEOLOGY • ANGELS • ASTROLOGY/
NUMEROLOGY • BIOGRAPHY/AUTOBIOGRAPHY
• BUDDHISM/ENLIGHTENMENT • BUSINESS/LEADERSHIP/
WISDOM • CELTIC/DRUID/PAGAN • CHANNELLING
• CHRISTIANITY; EARLY • CHRISTIANITY; TRADITIONAL
• CHRISTIANITY; PROGRESSIVE • CHRISTIANITY;
DEVOTIONAL • CHILDREN'S SPIRITUALITY • CHILDREN'S
BIBLE STORIES • CHILDREN'S BOARD/NOVELTY • CREATIVE
SPIRITUALITY • CURRENT AFFAIRS/RELIGIOUS • ECONOMY/
POLITICS/SUSTAINABILITY • ENVIRONMENT/EARTH
• FICTION • GODDESS/FEMININE • HEALTH/FITNESS
• HEALING/REIKI • HINDUISM/ADVAITA/VEDANTA
• HISTORY/ARCHAEOLOGY • HOLISTIC SPIRITUALITY
• INTERFAITH/ECUMENICAL • ISLAM/SUFISM
• JUDAISM/CHRISTIANITY • MEDITATION/PRAYER
• MYSTERY/PARANORMAL • MYSTICISM • MYTHS
• POETRY • RELATIONSHIPS/LOVE • RELIGION/
PHILOSOPHY • SCHOOL TITLES • SCIENCE/
RELIGION • SELF-HELP/PSYCHOLOGY
• SPIRITUAL SEARCH • WORLD
RELIGIONS/SCRIPTURES • YOGA

Please visit our website,
www.O-books.net